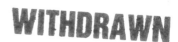

THE
EASY STRETCHING
WORKBOOK

THE EASY STRETCHING WORKBOOK

KAREN SMITH

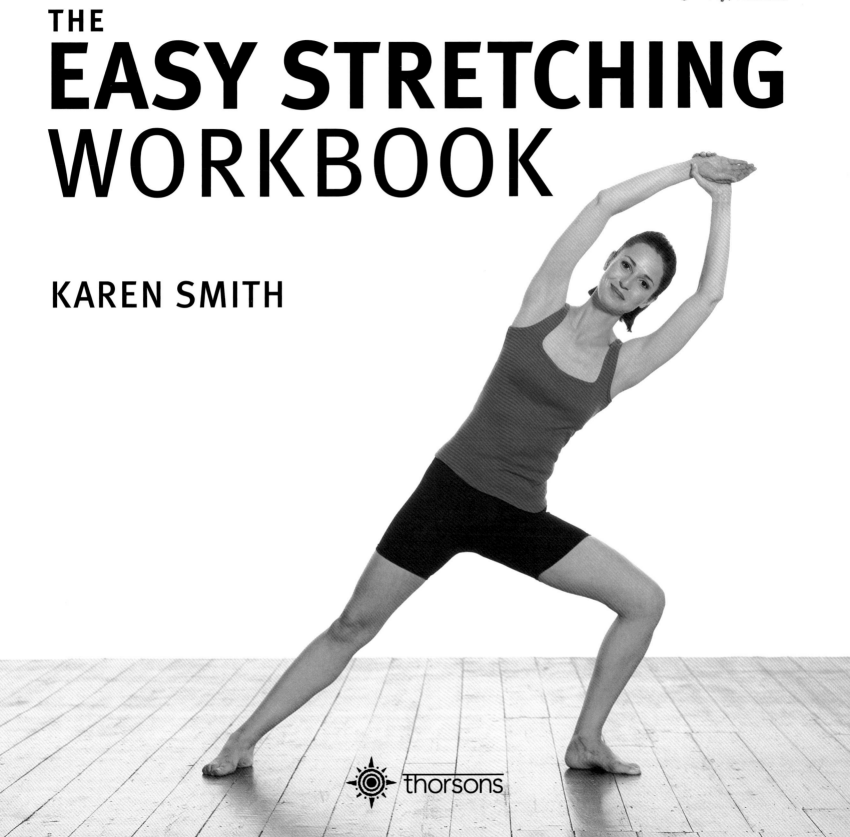

thorsons

The Easy Stretching Workbook
Karen Smith

Thorsons
An Imprint of HarperCollins*Publishers*
77–85 Fulham Palace Road
Hammersmith, London W6 8JB

The website address is: www.thorsonselement.com

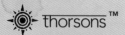

and *Thorsons* are trademarks of HarperCollins*Publishers* Ltd

First published in the US by Thorsons 2004

10 9 8 7 6 5 4 3 2 1

Conceived, created, and designed by Duncan Baird Publishers Ltd

Copyright © Duncan Baird Publishers 2004
Text copyright © Karen Smith 2004
Copyright of photographs © Duncan Baird Publishers 2004

Karen Smith asserts the moral right to be identified as the author
of this work.

Cataloging-in Publication Data is available from the
Library of Congress

ISBN: 0-00-769581-0

Color reproduction by Color & Print Gallery Sdn Bhd, Malaysia
Printed in China by Imago

NOTES
Before following any advice or practice suggested in this book,
it is recommended that you consult your doctor as to its suitability,
especially if you suffer from any health problems or special
conditions. The publisher, the author, and the photographer cannot
accept any responsibility for any injuries or damage incurred as
a result of following the exercises in this book, or of using any
of the therapeutic techniques described or mentioned here.

For my pupils of dance and Pilates –
you are my learning curve.

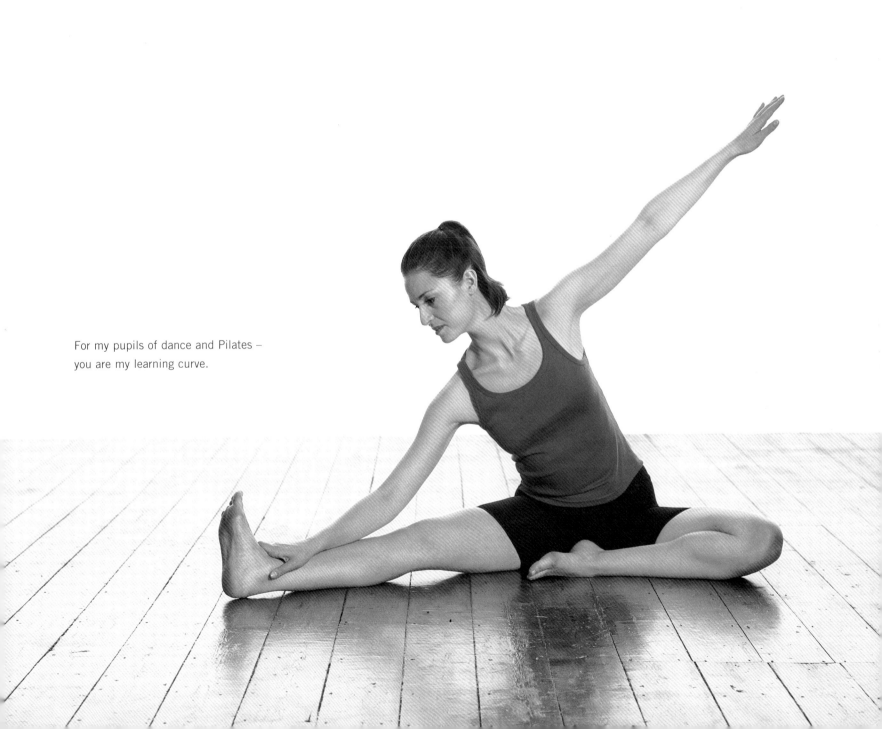

Contents

SYMBOLS USED IN THIS BOOK

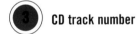 CD track number

✓ Stretch is good for ... / Solution to problem

✗ Avoid if ... / Problem with stretch

❗ Take care if you suffer from ...

◎ See Chapter 3 for troubleshooting tips

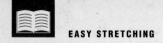

Author's introduction

I have been stretching for as long as I can remember. At the age of three I began taking ballet lessons, and went on to train seriously, finally becoming a professional dancer. During my career I sometimes woke up aching all over – a direct result of the previous day's gruelling performance. However, I discovered that when I practised some basic stretches prior to rehearsals and performances, my pain would diminish. This demonstrates how stretching can help the human body to recover, even when it has been pushed to its limits.

Unfortunately my career was cut short by a serious car accident, in which I broke my neck and became completely paralyzed. I lay in hospital for three months, attempting to stretch my wasted muscles and eventually recovered enough to walk again. From this experience I learned that where there is life in the body, there is the ability to stretch.

It is not just dancers, athletes and sports people who need to stretch. We all do, regardless of age and ability. Once you begin to stretch and discover more about your body, you will soon realize that stretching offers many benefits.

I am still learning about the process of stretching from teaching ballet and Pilates. Every day in my classes I meet people, each of whom has different physical needs. Throughout their lives those people's needs will alter, either because of changing circumstances or the ageing process. But if they keep stretching, they will stay in shape and enjoy good health. As I tell my students – if you want to extend your life, start extending your body!

How to use this book

This book contains photographs, a CD and all the information you need to build up a simple stretching routine in the comfort of your own home. Before you start exercising I suggest that you first read How to Stretch Safely (pp.19–20), How Not to Stretch (p.21) and Warm-up Exercises (pp.22–3) as they offer useful advice.

Chapter 1 outlines the benefits of stretching and explains how our muscles work – particularly those in the spine, the shoulders and the hamstrings.

Chapter 2 shows twenty step-by-step stretches for different areas of the body.

Chapter 3 suggests alternative or modified versions of the stretches in Chapter 2, which you will find particularly useful if you are experiencing any difficulties with these exercises.

Chapter 4 explores methods of relaxation. These can be practised separately or incorporated into your program after the stretches.

Chapter 5 guides you through stretches that are beneficial if you play certain sports, such as soccer, or if you take part in activities, such as aerobics.

Finally, Chapter 6 helps you to combat the stress and strain we all suffer through modern lifestyles, offering stretches to help you perform every day tasks as well as stretches to do when travelling.

The CD features audio instructions for each stretch in Chapter 2, and is intended to complement the book. Always look at the photographs and read the text in the book before commencing, so that you can visualize the target positions for the stretches while you listen to the instructions.

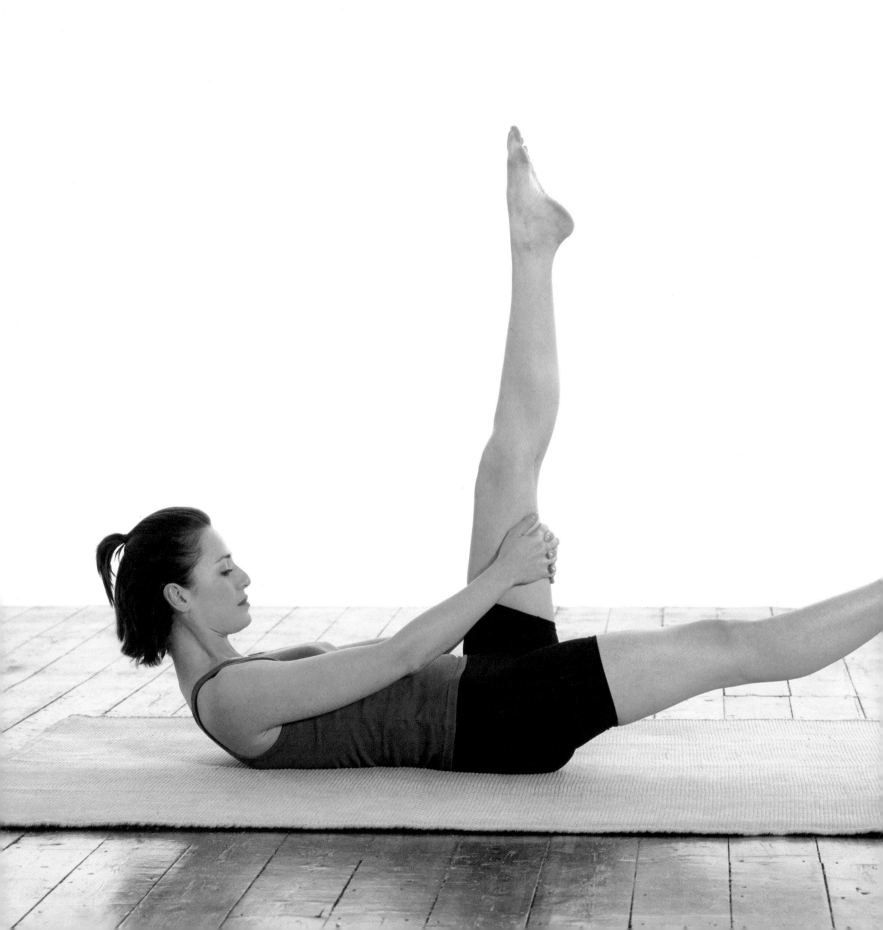

CHAPTER 1:
Easy Principles

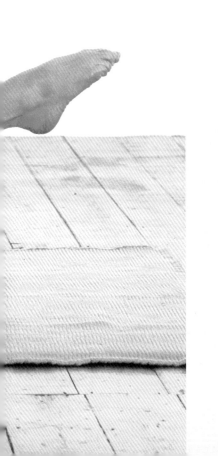

Stretching should never be a stressful activity – it should be relaxing and non-competitive. You don't need to be physically fit to start stretching. Even if you have never exercised before or you haven't exercised for a long time, stretching will allow you to get in touch with your muscles and improve your body's flexibility.

To gain maximum benefit from stretching, tailor your workout to suit your personal needs and your own musculature. If you practise as often as you can, stretching will gradually become an integral part of your lifestyle. Whatever your age, you will benefit from feeling healthier and finding life more rewarding.

Whether you sit at a desk all day, do physical work or drive long distances, this chapter will give you all the information you need to enable you to stretch safely and enjoyably.

Why stretch?

Our ancestors did not suffer the same physical problems that we have today. They did hard physical work just to survive. During the Industrial Revolution machines that saved time and labour were invented, but these same machines have made us more sedentary, which has created problems for our bodies. For example, we now often drive instead of walking and we use escalators or elevators instead of stairs. With no natural physical outlets for our daily tension, our muscles become weaker and less flexible and our joints come under more strain.

The skeleton, which forms the main structure of our body, needs a lot of support from our muscles. When the muscles are stretched regularly they become more elastic, giving the joints a wider range of movement. This flexibility in the joints prevents the body from seizing up and becoming stiff. And, a flexible, stretched muscle resists stress far better than a stiff, unstretched muscle.

You will not find a more intricate and superb mechanism than the human body, but these days we rarely allow our bodies to function in the way that they were designed to. Constant compression of the spine and the joints causes wear and tear, and can result in disc degeneration or serious conditions such as arthritis and osteoporosis. Stretching can help you to take the weight off your spine and release the tension in the joints.

Many of you are probably walking around with a constant feeling of stiffness in certain muscles – they have become like tight elastic bands pulling on your joints. If you are not used to stretching or exercising you will be unaware that this feeling is anything unusual. You may notice that you have a little neck and shoulder tension, but choose to ignore it. Carrying so much tension in the body actually puts quite a strain on it, and also makes you feel tired. When you stretch your muscles, they receive more nourishment from the blood, so your whole body feels healthier and more energized.

The other benefits of stretching include improving your coordination by allowing freer and easier movements, and correcting your posture, as longer, stretched muscles will make you stand straighter and taller. Stretching can also prevent injuries, such as muscle strains. And if you run, swim, ski, cycle or play tennis or golf, stretching before performing your sport will prepare your body safely for activity and can also improve your performance.

Stretching is also a great way to get to know yourself physically – your awareness and knowledge of your body will increase as you focus on the different parts of it.

When you start stretching regularly you will soon notice the multiple benefits – as well as feeling more supple, you will also look younger and be happier!

The musculo-skeletal system

The diagram on the page opposite shows the main skeletal muscles. There are over six hundred of these in the human body, overlapping each other in convoluted layers. A skeletal muscle generally attaches to the end of one bone and stretches across a joint to attach to another bone. The muscles that are located just below the skin are known as the *superficial* muscles, and beneath these lie the *deep* muscles.

The neck muscles and the large triangular muscles of the upper back help to stabilize the head and shoulders and assist their complex range of movements. The most powerful muscles in the body are those either side of the spinal column. They help to maintain good posture and create strength for movements such as lifting and pushing. The skeletal muscles make up nearly half the total weight of the human body.

Muscles work in groups, stretching or contracting in response to nerve impulses and they can usually be controlled voluntarily. The muscle that contracts to produce movement is called the *agonist*, while its opposite, the relaxing muscle which lies on the other side of the joint, is known as the *antagonist*.

To make sure that your body is balanced correctly, it is a good idea to do the stretches for each area, even if some parts do not feel as stiff as others.

THE STRUCTURE AND FUNCTION OF A MUSCLE

There are three types of muscle: skeletal, smooth and cardiac, but for the purposes of stretching we are concerned only with the skeletal muscles. These are composed of bundles of long, striated fibres, held together with connective tissue. Numerous capillaries penetrate this tissue to supply it with oxygen and glucose. Muscle fibres are surrounded by membranes and the bundles of fibres are encased in a sheath, rather like wires within a cable. The muscle membranes stretch along the whole length of the muscle from tendons located at both ends. The tendons link the skeletal muscles to the bones and ligaments hold the joints in position.

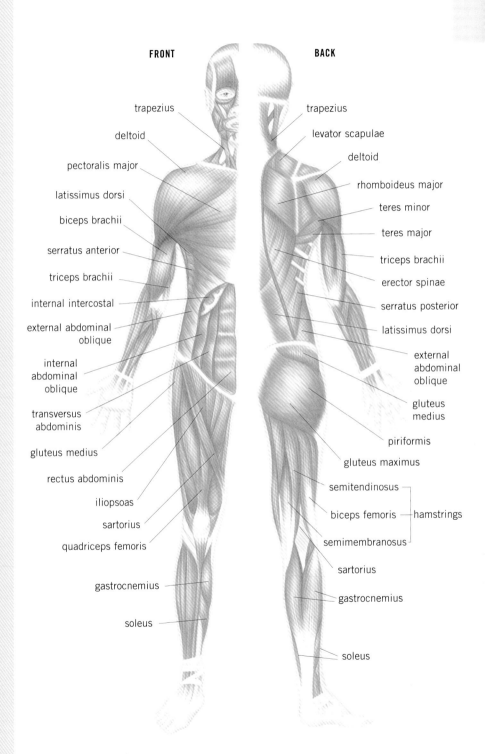

FRONT

trapezius
deltoid
pectoralis major
latissimus dorsi
biceps brachii
serratus anterior
triceps brachii
internal intercostal
external abdominal oblique
internal abdominal oblique
transversus abdominis
gluteus medius
rectus abdominis
iliopsoas
sartorius
quadriceps femoris
gastrocnemius
soleus

BACK

trapezius
levator scapulae
deltoid
rhomboideus major
teres minor
teres major
triceps brachii
erector spinae
serratus posterior
latissimus dorsi
external abdominal oblique
gluteus medius
piriformis
gluteus maximus
semitendinosus ⎤
biceps femoris ⎬ hamstrings
semimembranosus ⎦
sartorius
gastrocnemius
soleus

THE SPINE

The spine is made up of 33 vertebrae, which are ring-like bones. There are three main types of vertebrae: cervical (in the neck), thoracic (in the upper and mid back) and lumbar (in the lower back). At the base of the spine lies the wedge-shaped sacrum and the coccyx, which is also known as the tailbone. There are cartilage discs between the vertebrae, which act as shock absorbers. Strong ligaments and muscles around the spine help to stabilize the vertebrae and control movement. The spinal cord extends from the brainstem down through the spinal column to the lower back. There are 31 pairs of spinal nerves, which radiate outward from the spinal cord between the

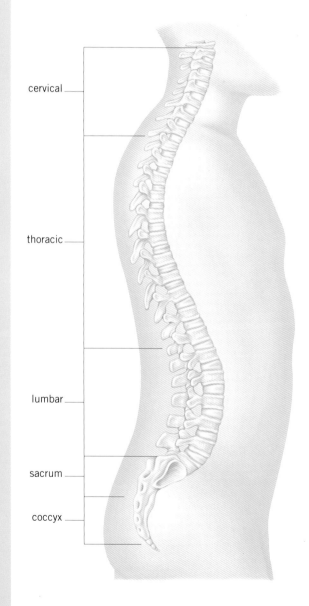

cervical

thoracic

lumbar

sacrum

coccyx

vertebral spaces and travel to the body tissues and organs.

A healthy spine should have four natural curves, which help us maintain our balance and provide flexibility. Sometimes we do not take good care of this precious part of our anatomy – many of us will suffer from back pain at some stage in our life. To maintain a healthy spine you need to move it often to relieve pressure from the discs and to relax your back muscles.

THE NECK AND SHOULDERS

Neck and shoulder pain is increasingly common. The weight of an average human head is between seven and ten pounds (3.15 and 4.5 kilos) and is supported by the structure and the muscles of the neck and shoulders.

The shoulder joint is one of the most complicated in the body. It acts both as a centre of movement and as a stabilizer for actions with the elbow, wrist and hand, having more range of movement than any other joint.

The shoulder relies heavily on its bones, ligaments and muscles for strength, stability and function. Its only bony attachment to the body is the collarbone. The rest of the shoulder girdle is held in position by a series of muscles. Two main groups of shoulder-stabilizing muscles help to maintain the position of the joint and move the shoulder in various directions. Some of them are connected to the arm bone.

I cannot overemphasize the importance of keeping your neck and shoulder muscles stretched and your joints mobilized. Keeping your neck flexible and free of tension is also crucial, as this area houses the top end of the main nerve pathway along which impulses from the brain and the spinal cord travel. Any restriction in the neck can affect the normal blood flow between these areas.

THE HAMSTRINGS

The hamstrings are the muscles that run from behind and below the knees, up the backs of the thighs to the "sitting-bones". There are actually three hamstring muscles on the back of each thigh: two on the inside and one on the outside. Today, because we spend so much time sitting, we do not stretch our hamstrings nearly enough. They are probably the longest, least-stretched muscles in the body.

The hamstrings have several functions. In addition to flexing and bending the knee, they also help to stabilize the knee during any twisting movement, such as turning a corner when walking or skiing.

Tight hamstrings can be a cause of painful knees and poor posture. If your hamstrings are short and tight, they will greatly restrict your flexibility and increase the risk of damage to your lower back. This on-going tension can have far-reaching effects on your movement, your balance and the health of your joints.

How to stretch safely

Stretching is easy to learn, but there is a correct way and an incorrect way to stretch. Unfortunately, many of us have been conditioned into thinking that there is "no gain without pain" and that the more exercise hurts, the more you get out of it. Stretching, when done correctly, should never be painful.

Be aware of your body while you are stretching. If you feel pain, your position is probably wrong. When you stretch correctly you will feel relaxed and able to focus on the muscles you are stretching, which will help you to sustain the movement. Your breathing will be slow and controlled — but never hold your breath for a long time. It is always helpful to exhale as you start the stretch so that the flow of the breath helps you to move with the flow of the movement. If you are stretching for the first time, or if you have not stretched for a while, it is a good idea to spend only a few seconds in each stretch position. On the other hand, if you are used to stretching, you can hold the positions for longer.

Regardless of whether you are new to stretching or not, it is *how* you stretch that is important. Inhale to prepare for each stretch, exhale as you go to the point where you feel mild tension and then try to relax while you hold the stretch. Keep breathing naturally and you should feel the tension ease slightly as you hold the position. If the tension does not subside, ease off a little until you feel more comfortable. Everyone is different physically and it is just a matter of finding the boundary between your comfort and pain zones. However, note that if you always stay within your comfort zone you will never increase your flexibility.

Never overstretch. If you stretch the muscle fibres too far, a nerve reflex responds by sending a signal to the muscles to contract, to protect them from injury. Therefore, stretching too far actually tightens the very muscles you are trying to relax!

WHEN TO STRETCH

Stretching can be done at any time, provided you are warm enough. If you stretch in the morning, your body will be more mobile during the rest of the day because you will have lengthened your muscles. This prepares your body for action. You can still carry on stretching throughout the day: at work to release nervous tension; after sitting or standing for any length of time; or whenever you feel stiff. You can even stretch while watching television, reading or listening to music in the evening. The key is to listen to your body – it will tell you when it needs to be stretched. You can learn a lot by observing a cat, an animal that instinctively knows when and how to stretch to tune up its muscles. A cat never overstretches – it stretches to prepare its muscles for the next movement.

How not to stretch

Stretching should never be practised in a fast jerky manner. A sudden, quick stretch does not allow the muscle to adapt and change length correctly, which can result in more tension building up.

You should be careful not to bounce when you stretch. "Ballistic" stretching, as this is known, can damage your muscles by causing micro-tears in the muscle fibres – especially if you haven't warmed up properly. Incorrect stretching can also damage the joints, particularly if your body is badly aligned. Forcing the stretch too far can overstretch the ligaments and also place a strain on your tendons. Flexibility without the strength to control it is likely to lead to injury. It is far better to have good strength and adequate flexibility than great flexibility and inappropriate weakness.

WHEN NOT TO STRETCH

Never stretch when your muscles are cold, or after you have sustained an injury. Inflammation usually occurs as part of the healing process and it is better to wait until this has resolved. Always allow at least an hour after a meal before stretching. If you have osteoporosis, arthritis or any other degenerative condition, it is best to seek advice from your doctor, physiotherapist or osteopath. Also consult your doctor before stretching if you are pregnant.

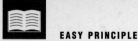

Warm-up exercises

Anyone who has ever taken part in a sport, or any form of exercise will be familiar with the concept of warming up before exercising. The reason why warming up is so important is because the body works more efficiently when warm – if you practise a sport and you forget or decide not to warm up, not only will your performance suffer, but you are also much more likely to injure yourself.

Warming up means raising your body temperature. When you are warm your body becomes more flexible without stretching. This is because the connective tissues, the muscles, the tendons and the ligaments become more pliable when they are warm. Normally, when our muscles are relaxed, only about fifteen per cent of the body's blood reaches them. The rest is channelled toward the vital organs, such as the brain, the intestines and the liver.

If you are doing vigorous exercise, your muscles will require almost eighty per cent of your blood to circulate through them to give them nourishment. You should never exercise nor embark on your exercise routine within an hour of eating a heavy meal. This is because, after you have eaten, your blood is needed for the process of digestion and therefore needs to remain in the stomach and intestines, rather than be diverted to the muscles. Also, if you exercise too soon after a meal you could suffer from stomach cramps.

In cold weather, you may need to do more work to warm up properly than you would need to do if the temperature was warm. The amount of warming up you require will also depend on your fitness level in general and whether you are embarking on a high-energy exercise program. For example, a warm-up before a game of football would need to be more extensive than a warm-up before a game of bowls.

Effective warm-up activities should be continuous and flowing, such as gentle jogging, fast walking, cycling or jumping on a mini-trampoline. If you can't do any of these, you could just walk as you usually do, or a little faster, and swing your arms vigorously for a few minutes. You can easily do this at home. Put on some music with a fast beat and march on the spot. When you raise your left knee, swing your right arm and vice versa. The higher you manage to swing your arms, the faster your heart will beat.

Remember, the aim of performing warm-up exercises is to increase your body temperature, which will make your muscles more flexible for your stretching session. To make this happen you need to increase your heart rate so that you get warm and feel slightly out of breath. Changes in your body's temperature will also vary according to your size, how much you weigh and your metabolic rate.

Practical basics

We all have a unique body shape and size, but the ideal physique is as strong and flexible as possible. Too much strength and not enough flexibility, or vice versa can lead to physical problems. The important thing is to have a balanced exercise routine. For example, if you go to the gym regularly, you probably concentrate on cardiovascular and strength training. If this describes you, you would benefit from including some stretching in your routine, to improve your flexibility. Or, if your lifestyle involves a lot of sitting, for example working at a computer all day, you would probably find the standing stretches helpful. On the other hand, if you tend to rush around rather a lot during a typical day or you have a job that entails standing, you might benefit most from the stretches that involve lying on the floor. And you would probably enjoy the relaxation exercises too!

If you have no energy, or have recently been ill, start with say, five stretches and gradually introduce more as you feel better.

In some of the stretches, I have suggested that you use a stretchband, as the resistance in the band helps you to stretch further. The bands are available in a variety of tensions, but it is advisable to start with a low-tension one. Where possible, I offer an alternative to the band, such as a scarf or a broomhandle, and I give at least one way to do each exercise without a band.

STRETCHING TIPS

Here are a few guidelines to help you feel comfortable and enjoy your stretching exercises more:

- Wear comfortable clothing that doesn't restrict your movement.

- Practise in a warm, ventilated room away from draughts.

- Use a small cushion or book to rest your head on if you feel discomfort at the back of your neck when lying down.

- Use a towel or an exercise mat to cushion your spine when lying down.

- Never stretch directly after a meal. Always leave at least an hour before stretching.

- Go into each stretch gently.

- Relax into your breathing. Inhale through your nose and exhale through your mouth.

- Focus on maintaining a strong "core" (see pp. 26–7) while stretching.

- Don't stretch too far too soon. You may not feel any discomfort at the time, but you might regret it the next day!

- Don't repeat the stretches too many times. Follow the guidelines, step by step.

- Come out of each stretch as gently as you went into it.

- When you begin stretching, don't expect your own position to match the target position.

- Stretch to help you improve in whatever you do in life.

Exercise basics

STRONG ABDOMINALS

One of the instructions I give throughout the stretches is to "keep your abdominals strong." If you have ever done Pilates, you will already know what this means. But for those of you who are unfamiliar with this term, it simply refers to maintaining a strong and stable abdominal centre while exercising, to support and protect your lower back.

Known as the "girdle of strength", a strong centre or "core" is extremely important if you wish to stretch correctly, because it enables you to move your limbs with more power and control. And unless you stabilize your core when stretching, your spine will be under stress and at risk of injury. The muscles used in creating and maintaining a strong centre are the pelvic floor muscles and the deep abdominal muscles, such as the *transversus abdominis* (see diagram, p.15), which also helps you to maintain good posture.

Creating a strong core does not mean tightly gripping your abdominals – this will only make the area more tense. Begin by drawing your pelvic floor muscles upward and hollowing out your lower abdominals by drawing them back toward your spine. Imagine you are wearing a corset that has been laced up around your middle. This is the support that you always need to feel around your abdomen, regardless of whichever area of your body you are stretching.

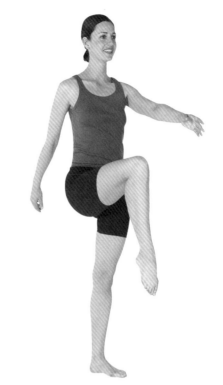

THE IMPORTANCE OF CORRECT POSTURE

Before you start stretching, make sure that you know how to stand with your body correctly aligned. Stand in front of a mirror with your feet parallel and hip-width apart, hands resting by your thighs. Stabilize your core and relax your shoulders. Now turn to the side and draw an imaginary straight line down through your body, from your ear to your ankle bone. If you are standing correctly, the two points will be exactly aligned.

PRIORITIZE YOUR STIFFER SIDE

Most of us have one side of the body that feels stiffer than the other when we stretch. For example, if you are right-handed you may find that you are tighter in your right shoulder and arm, and in the right sides of your neck and upper spine. This is simply because you use the muscles on the right side of your body more and they are stronger. The same applies to the left side, if you are left-handed.

In many people, the strength in their dominant side causes tension. For this reason I recommend that you practise stretches an extra two or three times on the tight side of your body, to release tension evenly on both sides.

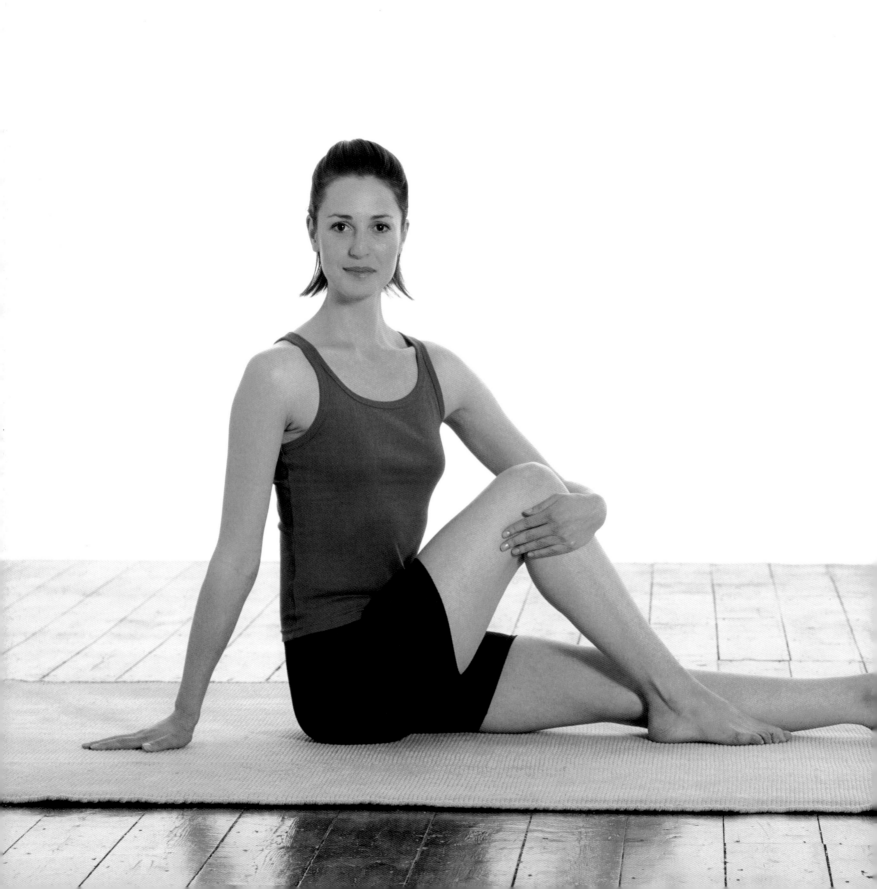

CHAPTER 2:
Easy Stretches

In this chapter there are twenty stretches. Each one is designed to stretch and mobilize a different area of the body and is illustrated in a photograph showing the correct stretching position. Don't worry if you are unable to attain these positions at first — as your body gets used to stretching, you will find them easier to achieve.

A word of caution — before attempting each stretch, please check the "avoid if ..." guidelines, which are given in the margin of each left-hand page, in case you have a condition that makes a particular stretch unsuitable. And, if you have difficulty doing any of the stretches, look in Chapter 3 to find out how you can modify the movement or do the stretch in a different, easier way.

Head tilt

GOOD FOR:

Easing tension in the
side of the neck and
the shoulders

SEE P.76

Stand on the middle of the stretchband with your feet hip-width apart. Hold the ends of the band in each hand, palms facing toward the sides of your hips. Keep your back straight and your abdominals strong. Focus straight ahead and breathe in. As you breathe out tilt your head toward your right shoulder. You will feel the left side of your neck stretch. Let your left shoulder drop. Breathe in and bring your head back to the starting position. Breathe out and repeat the movements to the other side. Repeat 4 or more times to each side.

NOTES

This stretch is more powerful than it looks, so don't stay in this position too long. Always use a light-tension band for any neck and shoulder stretches. Pulling against the resistance of the band makes you feel more length through the neck and arms. Relax your shoulders. If you can do this in front of a mirror, it will help you to tilt your head correctly sideways rather than turn it or tilt it backward. Focus on yourself in the mirror as you tilt your head gently toward the top of your shoulder. Use your breath to guide you through the movement. Keep your knees slightly soft as locking them into a rigid position could push your hips back.

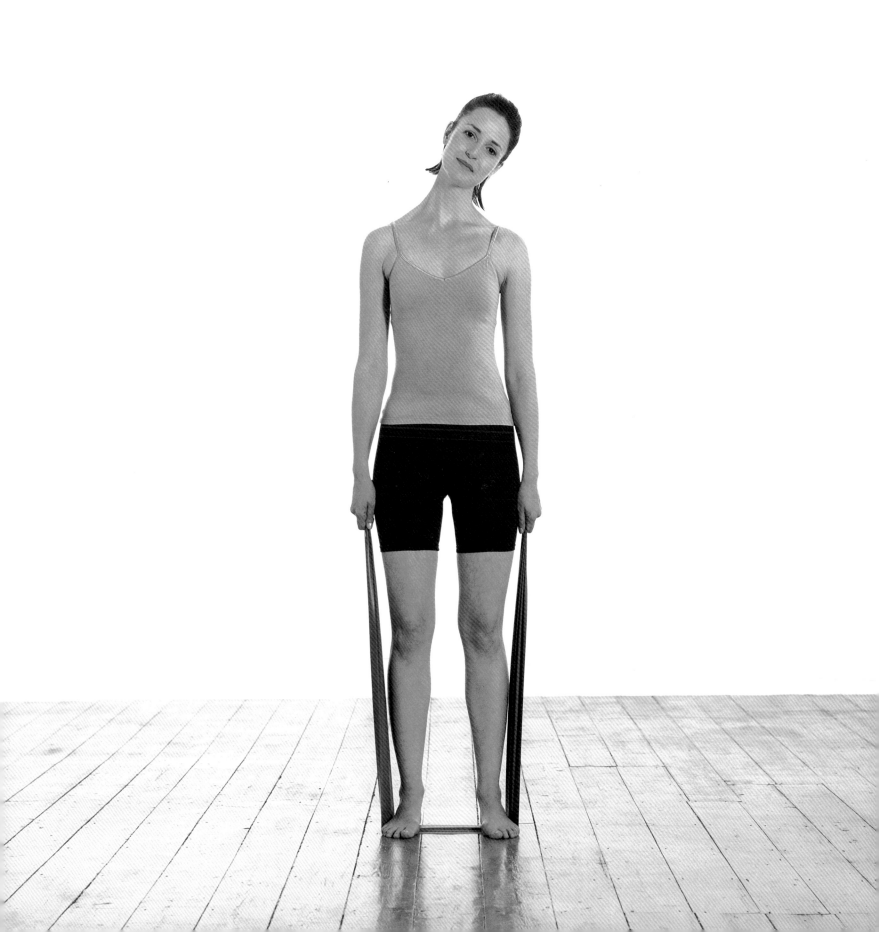

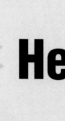

Head nod

(3)

 GOOD FOR:

Easing tension at the back of the neck and in the upper back

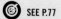 **SEE P.77**

Stand on the centre of the stretchband with your feet hip-width apart. Hold each end of the band with your palms facing toward the hips. Relax your shoulders so that your spine feels long. Breathe in and feel yourself growing a little taller, upward from the top of your head. Breathe out and nod your head down toward your chest. Make sure that you don't force your head too far forward. Feel the stretch down the back of your neck and between your shoulders. Breathe in and bring your head back up. Repeat 4 more times.

NOTES

As with the head tilt, this is a deceptively strong stretch and you should be careful not to overstretch your neck. Keep your shoulders relaxed and dropped, and ensure that you don't pull them forward as you nod your head forward. You can also do this stretch tilting your head slightly backward. Again, be careful not to overstretch. Lift your chin slightly so that you can feel the stretch under it and in the front of your neck. As you do this stretch, try to maintain a strong abdominal centre and a straight, plumb-line posture from the top of your head to the tip of your tailbone.

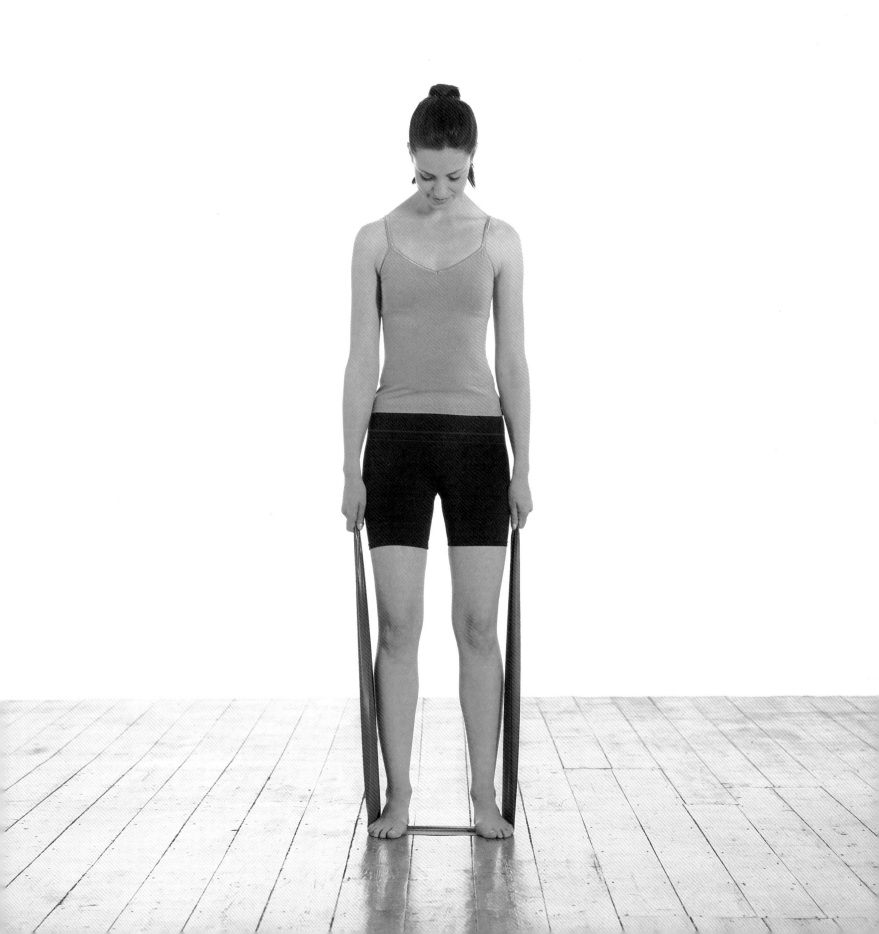

Shoulder release

(4)

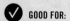 GOOD FOR:

Releasing neck and

shoulder tension

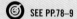 SEE PP.78–9

Stand on the centre of the stretchband with your feet hip-width apart. Hold each end of the band with your palms facing toward your hips. Keeping your knees soft, breathe in and raise your shoulders upward toward your ears. As you exhale slide your shoulders down again. Now extend your arms down toward the outsides of your knees. The sides of your neck should also feel longer as you stretch. Keep the movement flowing, as any jerky actions could cause tension. Repeat 5 to 8 times.

NOTES

Having a tense neck and shoulders is a common symptom of stress that office workers, in particular, often suffer from. This exercise aims to release that tension by isolating the shoulders from the rest of the body. When performing this stretch keep your spine straight and your abdominals strong. To vary the stretch you may like to add a circular movement with your shoulders: pull them slightly forward, then lift them up; pull them back and then slide them down. Now repeat the movement in reverse. This sequence of actions really increases mobility in the shoulder joints and helps to open out the upper back and chest.

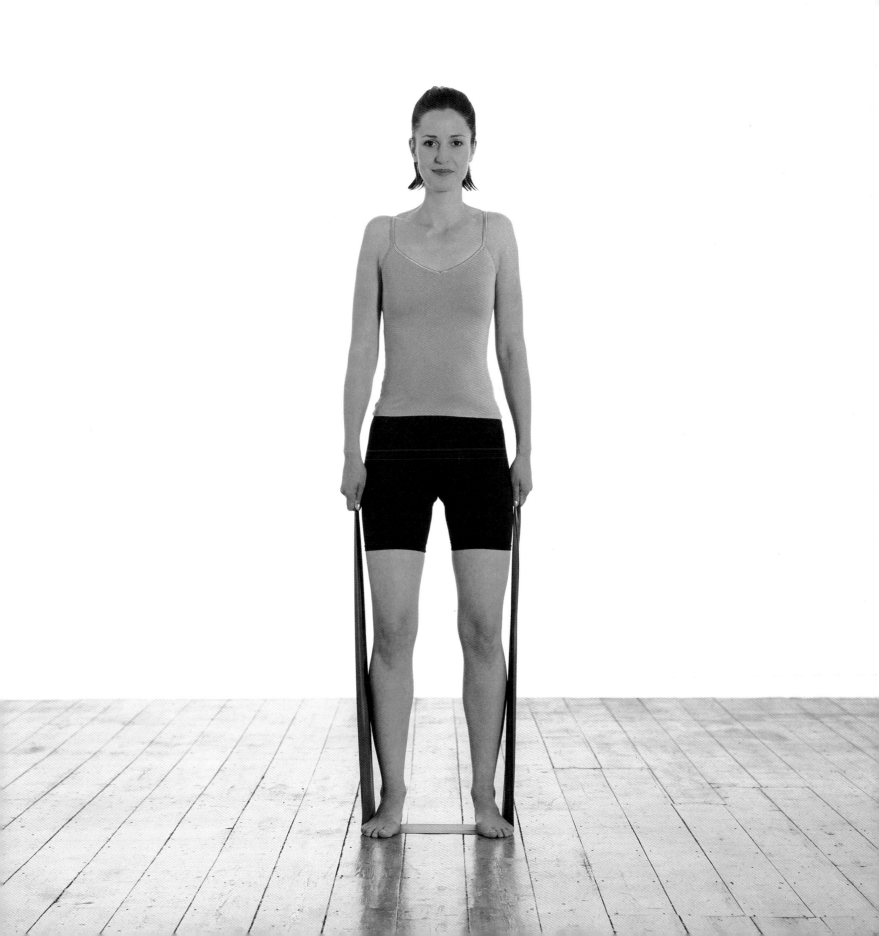

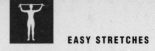

Upper chest and shoulder stretch

⑤

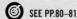 **GOOD FOR:**

Releasing tight shoulders and improving bad posture from sitting in front of a computer

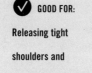 **SEE PP.80—81**

Stand with your feet hip-width apart. Hold the band in front of your body, your arms outstretched slightly wider than shoulder-width. Breathe in and lift up your arms above your head without raising your shoulders. As you exhale, stretch the band and bend your elbows as you pull the band down behind your shoulders. Be careful not to arch your back, or to stick your chin forward. Breathe in as you lift your arms up over your head, then exhale as you bring your arms back down to the starting position. Repeat 4 to 8 times.

NOTES

You will feel this stretch across the front of your shoulders and your upper chest. If you are very tight across the shoulders, try holding the band with your arms further apart. This will make it a little easier by lessening the resistance. As your chest and shoulders loosen up, you will be able to bring your arms closer together. Keep the rest of your body as still as possible and your stomach pulled in to prevent your lower back from arching and your hips from pushing forward. Also, keep your elbows slightly relaxed.

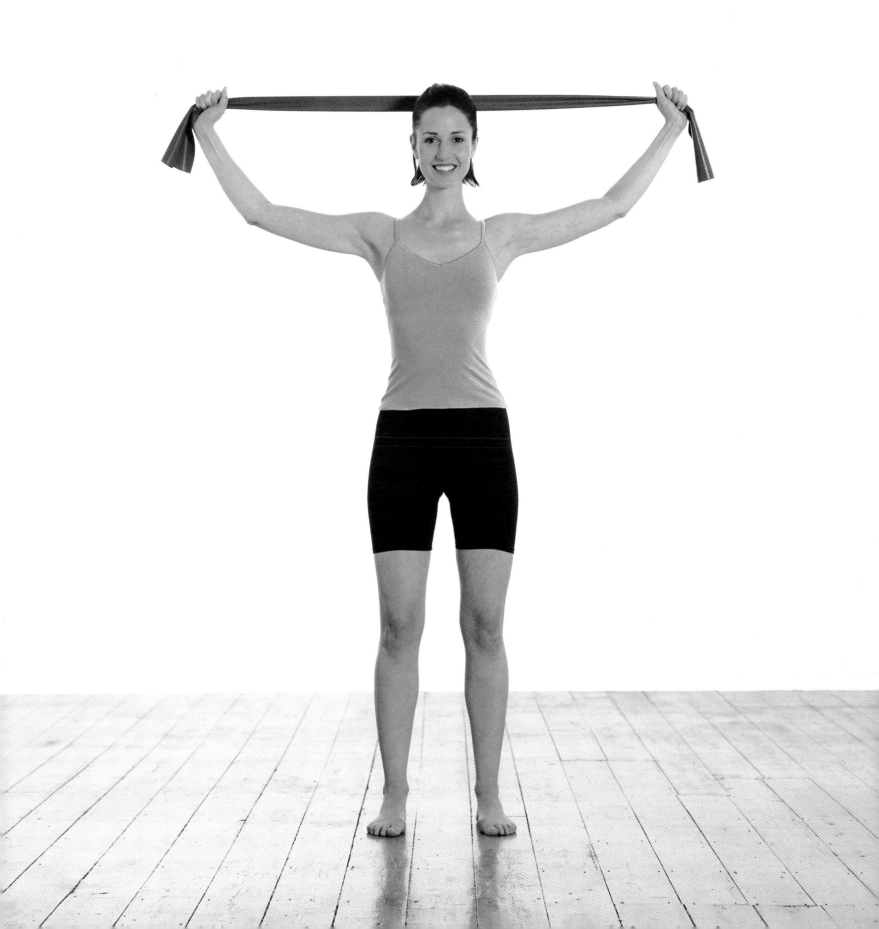

Upper arm and shoulder pull

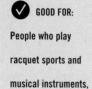 **GOOD FOR:**
People who play racquet sports and musical instruments, and those who use computer keyboards

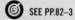 SEE PP.82–3

Stand with your feet hip-width apart. Stretch your arms out in front of you at just below shoulder height. Clasp your hands with your palms facing away from you. Inhale. As you exhale stretch your arms upward toward the ceiling – you should try to get your palms flat. Keep your shoulders down and your abdomen strong, and don't lock your elbows too rigidly. You should be able to feel the stretch all the way up your arms. Breathe in again, bend your elbows and bring your hands down toward your head. Repeat 4 more times.

NOTES

This is a good "wake-up" stretch to perform first thing in the morning. You can do it while still lying in bed. When you perform the stretch in a standing position, keep your eyes focused in front of you. As you reach up with your arms, try to feel that your waist is lengthening. As you exhale the first time, draw your abdominal muscles inward and try to maintain a strong centre throughout the exercise.

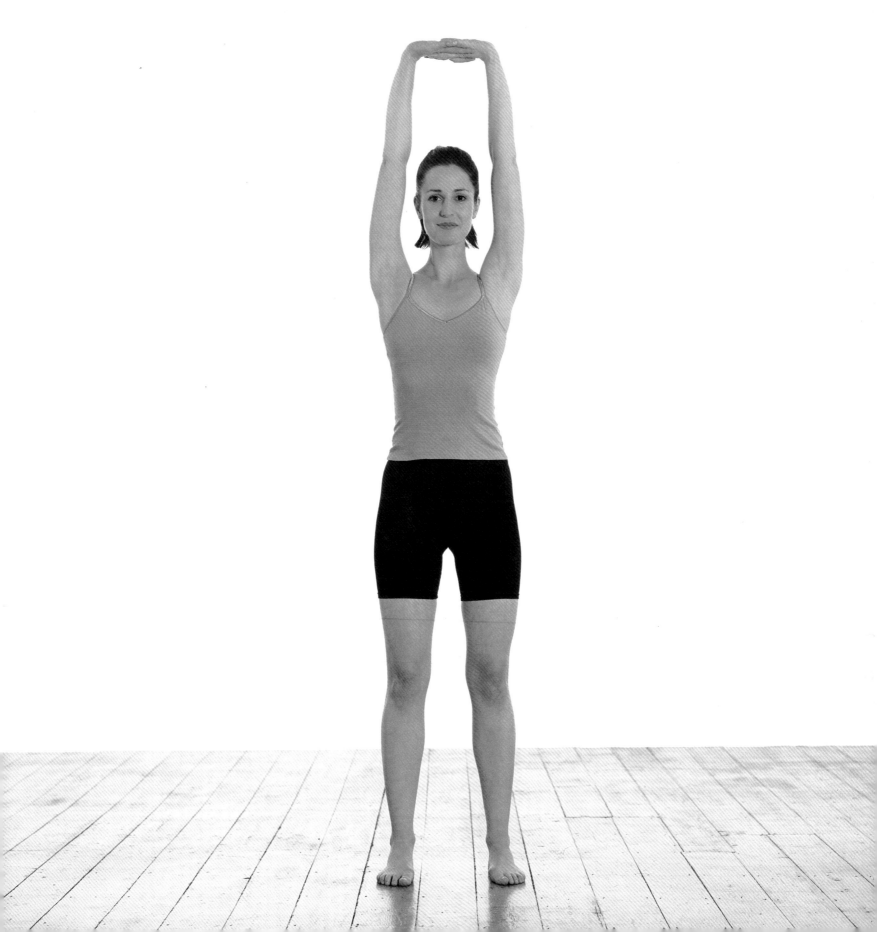

Spine twist

(7)

 GOOD FOR:
Opening out the
chest and shoulders,
stretching the
piriformis muscle and
mobilizing the spine

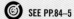 SEE PP.84–5

Sit on the floor with your left leg straight in front of you and your right knee bent. Rest your right foot alongside your left calf. Try to sit up as straight as possible, with your hands resting on the floor. Breathe in and place your left hand across your right knee, and as you exhale pull in your abdominals and twist your spine to the right. Feel your spine becoming longer and your shoulders pulling down. Turn your head to the right and feel your right shoulder opening out. Breathe in and relax your spine slightly, then breathe out and twist your spine again. Repeat 3 more times and then 5 times to the left side.

NOTES

Spinal rotation is important for maintaining a healthy back. However, it is extremely important to protect the spine from arching too much, by drawing in the abdominals. This stretch will also open out the chest and shoulders. Use the hand that is holding the knee to help you carry out the movement. Aim to keep your hips still as you twist your torso. Try to sit up straight on your "sitting-bones", and pull up from the hips – this will also help to stretch your lower back.

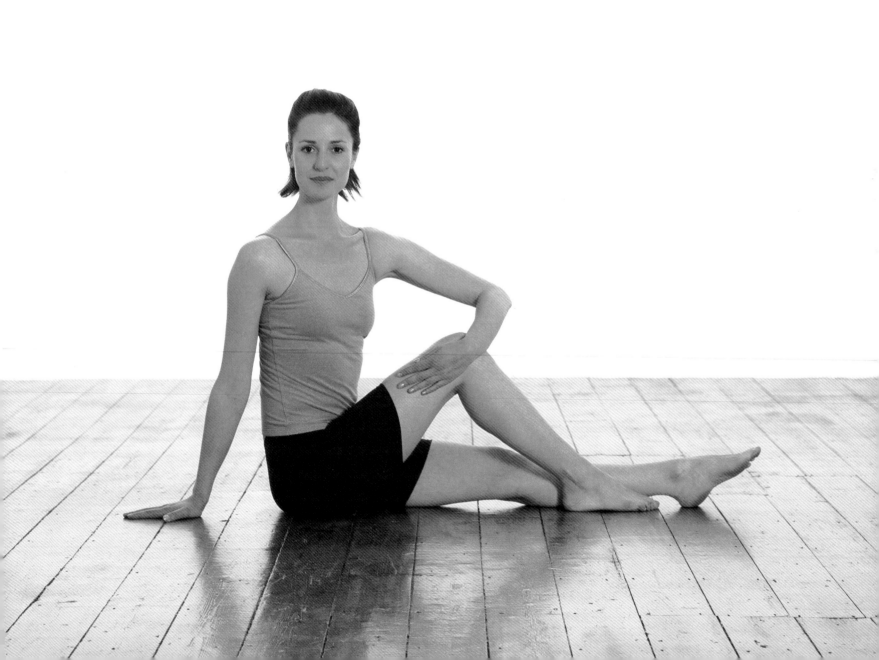

Spine stretch forward

GOOD FOR:

Relieving tightness
in the spine

TAKE CARE IF:

You have disc
problems or
osteoporosis
in the spine

SEE P.86

Stand with your knees slightly bent. Breathe in. As you breathe out slowly draw your abdominals in toward your lower spine. Drop your head gently forward – the weight of your head will make your spine roll down, vertebra by vertebra. Your head and arms should be hanging loosely and your stomach and ribs should be pulled in. Breathe in as you hold this position. Breathe out and, starting from the bottom of your spine, gradually uncurl your back upward, vertebra by vertebra, until your spine is straight again.

NOTES

This movement gently stretches the spine and opens out the spaces in between the vertebrae. It may help you to imagine that each vertebra is a spoke in a wheel as you roll your spine first down and then back up again. Relax your head, shoulders and arms completely on the way down. Keep your head and arms relaxed on the way back up, but pull your shoulders down. If your lower back feels tight, try tucking your hips under slightly as you uncurl your spine again. Keep your abdominals strong throughout this stretch.

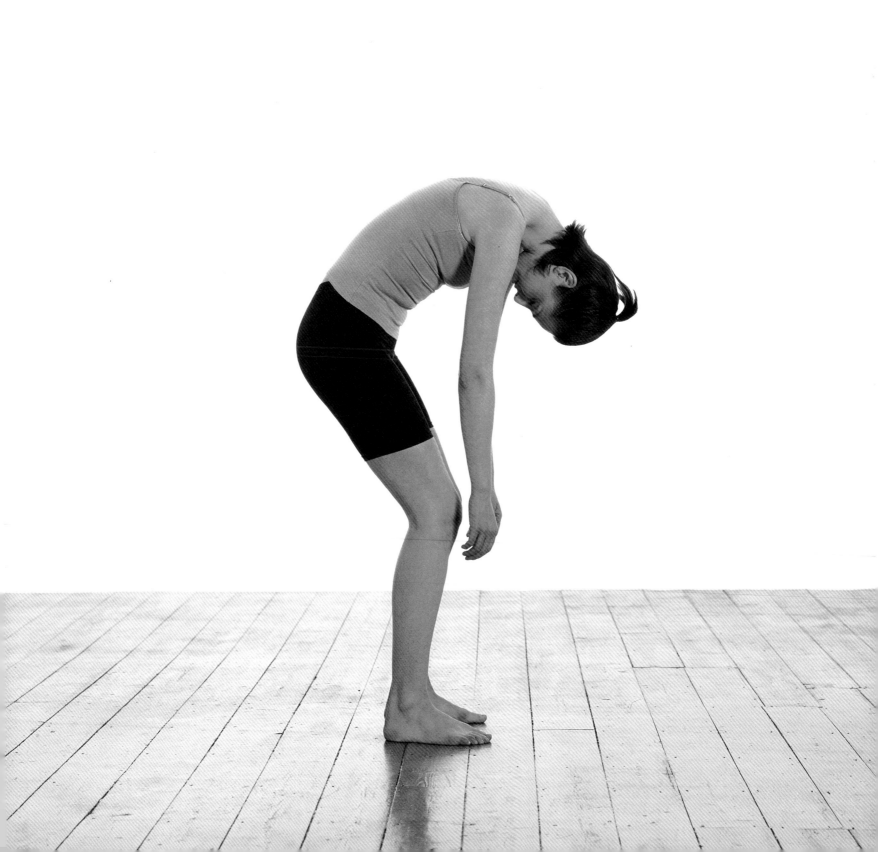

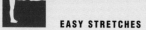

Spine stretch back

(9)

GOOD FOR:
Correcting bad posture from sitting at a desk and for releasing tightness in the upper chest

 SEE P.87

For this stretch you need a strong chair to lean upon. Stand facing the back of the chair with your arms extended in front of you at waist height. Your legs should be straight and your feet slightly wider than hip-width apart. Breathe in. Breathe out and lean forward so that your hands grasp the back of the chair. Bend forward from the waist and pull your shoulders down toward the back of your rib cage, keeping your knees slightly relaxed. Breathe in. Exhale and feel your whole spine lengthening as you lean further forward and stretch your back as much as you can. Repeat 3 times.

NOTES

This stretch opens out the upper spine and the area at the back of the shoulders. Aim to keep your back as long as possible from head to tailbone. Draw your abdominal muscles upward toward your lower spine and try to get the feeling of your upper chest reaching down toward the floor. If you want to incorporate a hamstring stretch into this exercise, you can straighten your knees without locking them too rigidly. Lengthen your tailbone as much as possible without arching your lower back.

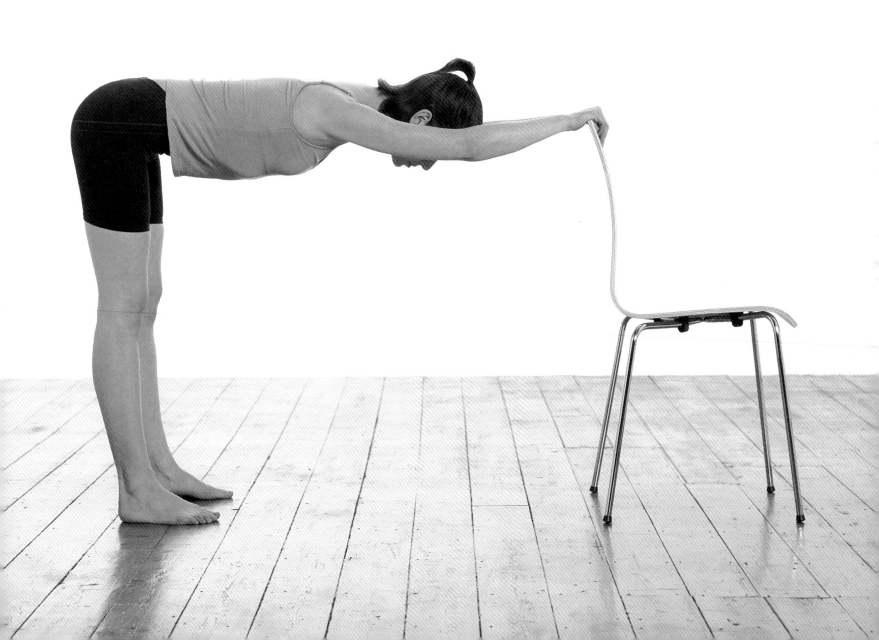

Chest curl

10

✔ **GOOD FOR:**
Strengthening the
abdominals

✘ **AVOID IF:**
You have osteoporosis
in the upper spine

◎ **SEE P.88**

Lie on your back with both knees bent, hip-width apart. Clasp your hands behind your head. Breathe in. Breathe out and curl your upper body away from the floor. Make sure that your hands support your head without pulling it. As you curl upward draw your abdominals in toward your lower spine, without moving your pelvis. Feel the tip of your tailbone touching the floor. Breathe in and roll back down — first your upper back, followed by your neck and then your head. Repeat 5 to 8 times.

NOTES

This stretch works the top part of the spine and the neck. Never pull the back of your head too vigorously as this could overstretch your neck. Your head should rest heavily in your hands. This is a wonderful exercise for strengthening the abdominal area, but the stretch is most beneficial if you practise it slowly with control, rather than quickly as "sit-ups". Keep your eyes focused on your knees. Always leave a little space between your chin and your upper chest. When performing this stretch it might help to imagine that there is a zip from your pubic bone to your navel and that each time you curl up you are doing it up.

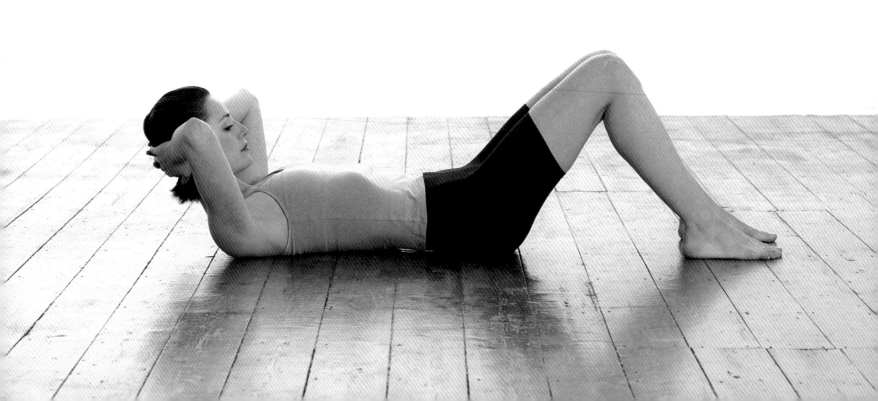

Kneeling back stretch

(11)

 GOOD FOR:
Opening the sacrum, stretching the whole spine and releasing the front of the hips

! TAKE CARE IF:
You have hip or knee replacements, or knee problems that affect the cartilage and ligaments

◎ SEE P.89

Start by sitting back on your heels, with your hands resting on your thighs. Breathe in. Exhale and lean forward from the hips stretching both your arms out in front of you on the floor. The aim is to rest your forehead on the floor while keeping your tailbone touching your heels. You may find this stretch easier if you open your knees slightly. Staying in this position, breathe in again and then exhale, drawing your abdominals in toward your lower spine. Reach out further with your arms, pull your shoulders down and try to lengthen your tailbone. Repeat 5 to 8 times.

NOTES

This is a wonderful back stretch – it releases and opens the sacrum. If you find it difficult to keep your tailbone in contact with your heels, try placing a cushion under your buttocks. You may also like to put a small cushion under your forehead. If your shoulders are uncomfortable, relax your arms by your sides. As you inhale you should feel your ribs widening. When coming out of this position, it is important to uncurl the bottom of the spine upward, so that your head is the last part to straighten up. Never sit bolt upright as this can strain the lower back.

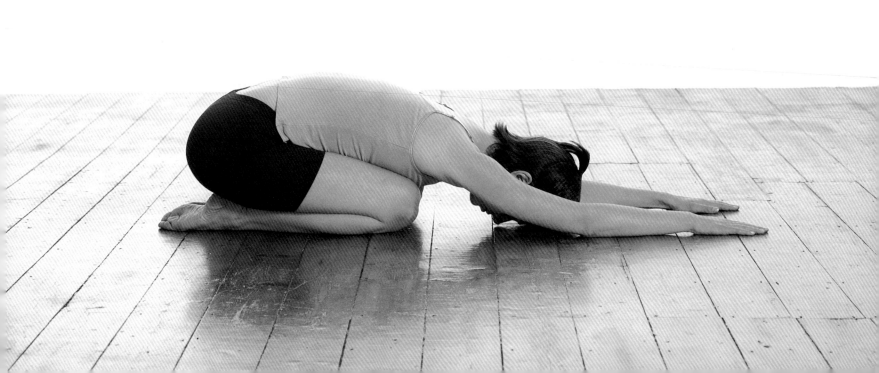

Waist stretch

(12)

GOOD FOR:
Reducing the waistline and stretching the lower spine

SEE PP.90–91

Stand with your feet hip-width apart. Hold on to the band with your arms outstretched a little wider than shoulder-width, at just below shoulder level. Breathe in. Lift your arms over your head, pull in your abdominals and lengthen your spine. As you exhale pull the left end of the band and bend sideways to the left. Use the resistance of the band to help you. You should feel a stretch along the right side of your waist. Breathe in as you straighten your spine. Repeat the stretch to the right side as you exale, this time pulling the right end of the band. Repeat 4 more times to each side.

NOTES

When doing this stretch be very careful not to move your hips, as this could place a strain on your lower back. As you bend to each side, pull both shoulders down. Don't twist your spine. Make sure that you keep your abdominals strong throughout. Each time you straighten your spine try to lengthen it a little more. This will enable you to reach further and extend the side stretch, which will soon improve your waistline!

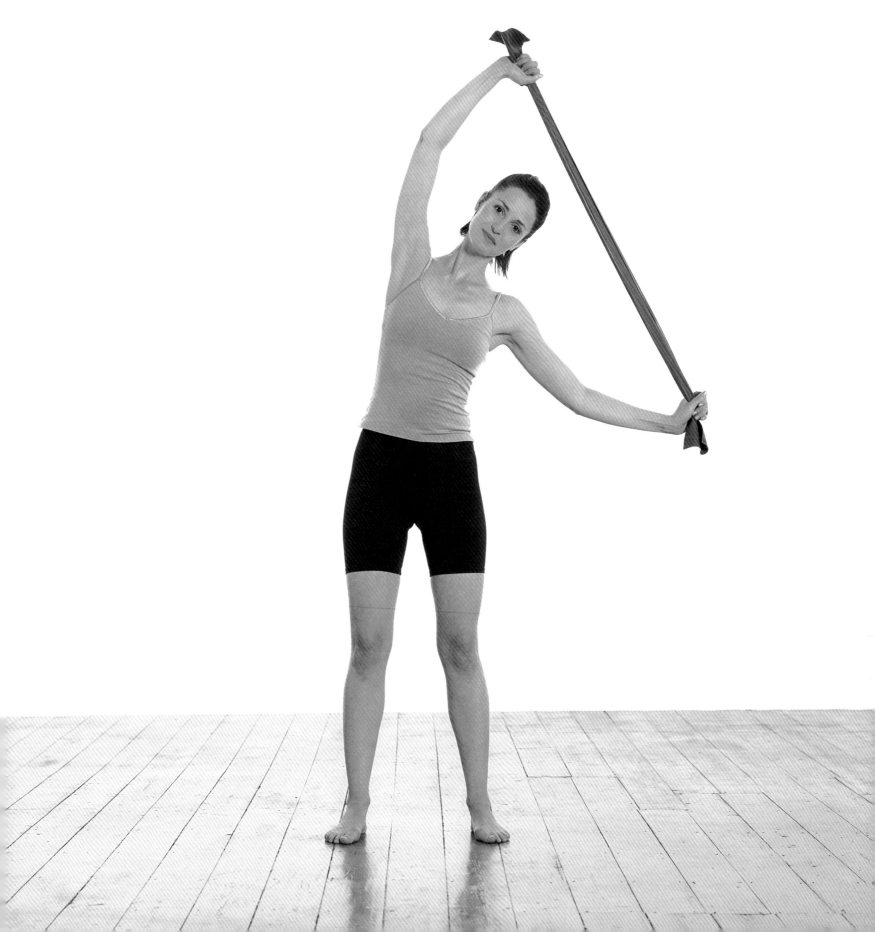

Front of hip stretch

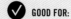

GOOD FOR:
Releasing tightness in the hip flexors, which is usually caused by too much sitting

 TAKE CARE IF:
You suffer from acute lower back pain

SEE P.92

At first you should practise this stretch holding on to a chair for support. Breathe in. As you exhale keep your back straight and slide your right leg behind you while bending your left leg. Keep your left knee directly over your left foot and most of your body weight on this leg. Allow the front of your right hip to sink forward and down. Keep the rest of your weight on the ball of your right foot. When you feel completely balanced, place both hands on your left knee. Stay in this position for a further four complete breaths. On each out-breath try to push your right heel back a little further. Repeat to the other side.

NOTES

This is a wonderful stretch for the front of the hip and the thigh. To help you hold your balance, keep your head lifted up and focus your eyes straight ahead. If your head drops you will be pulled forward. Keep your abdominals strong and your shoulders down. To come out of the stretch and to change legs, you can either place both your hands on the floor as you bend your back leg in, or you can rest them again on the back of the chair. Be sure to keep your abdominals strong when you change position.

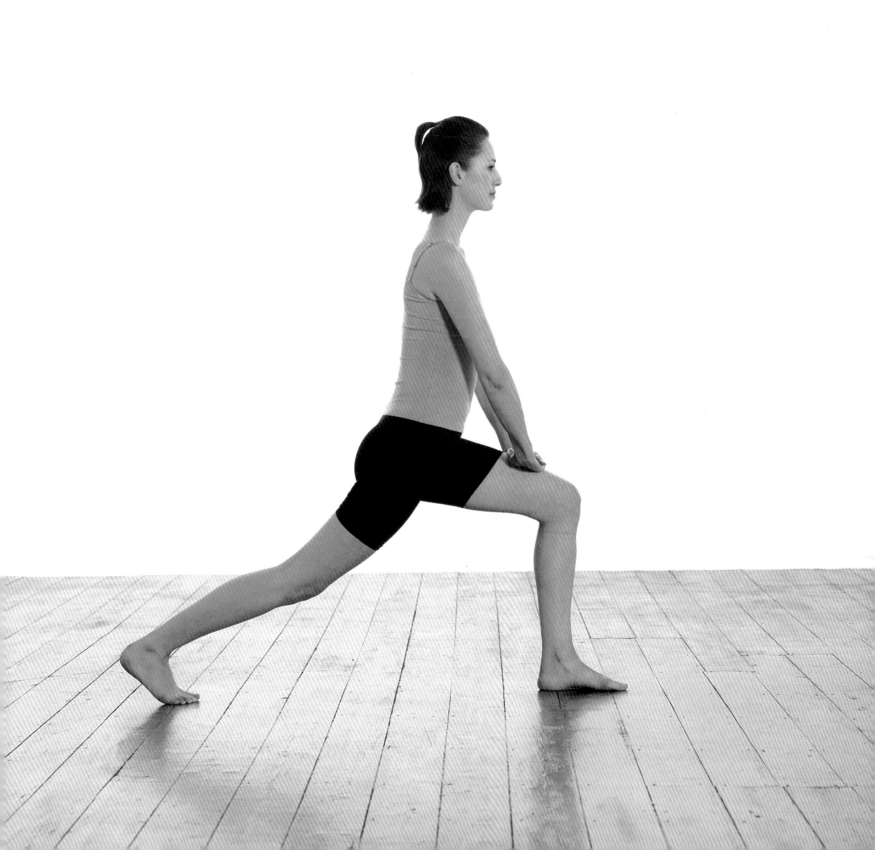

Side of hip stretch

14

GOOD FOR:
Stretching the side
of the hip and the
lower back

TAKE CARE IF:
You have hip
replacements

SEE P. 93

Lie on your back with both knees bent, arms down by your side. Cross your right leg over your left leg, as if you were sitting cross-legged. Breathe in. Exhale, draw your abdominals in strongly and roll your hips to your left. As you roll, gently turn your head to the right and try to relax both shoulders. Breathe in again. Exhale and engage your abdominal muscles more and let gravity pull your right knee down further. Keep your spine long. Stay in this position for three more breaths. Repeat with the left leg crossed, rolling to the right.

NOTES

This is a very good stretch for anyone who suffers with sciatica, or lower back or hip tightness. Try to maintain a feeling of length from the neck to the tailbone. If your back arches, it could be that your abdominal muscles aren't engaging enough. Focus on your core strength throughout the exercise, and particularly when bringing your hips back to the starting position to change legs. When rolling to the left, be careful that your right shoulder stays relaxed and vice versa. If you are very tight in the hips you may prefer to roll your hips over and rest your knees on a cushion.

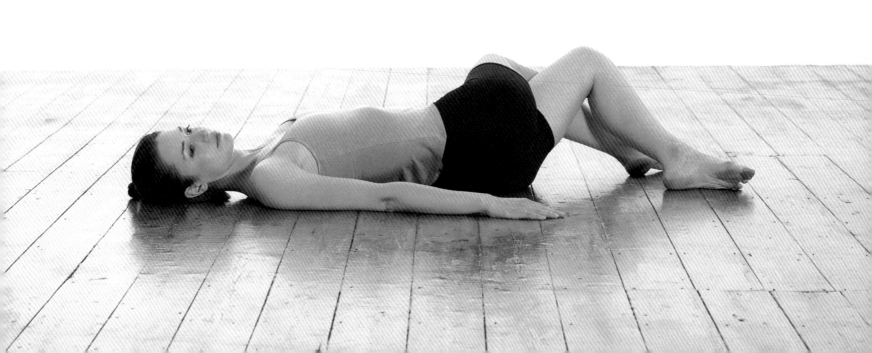

Buttock stretch

(15)

 GOOD FOR:
Releasing tightness
in the hips, the
piriformis muscle
and the gluteals
(the muscles in
the buttocks)

◎ SEE PP.94–5

Lie on the floor on your back, both knees bent, feet hip-width apart. Place your right ankle across the front of your left thigh, opening your right knee. Lift your left foot off the floor and place your right arm through the middle of both legs to clasp your hands at the back of your left thigh. Breathe in. As you exhale gently pull your left leg toward your chest. Use your right elbow as a lever to push the right knee open slightly. This will increase the stretch through the right buttock and open out your right hip. Repeat 5 to 8 times with each leg.

NOTES

This is a great stretch for anyone who suffers with sciatica, or lower back or hip tightness. Go gently at first as this exercise does provide quite a deep buttock stretch. If you have knee problems, you can do this stretch by crossing your legs while keeping your thighs together. Lift both feet off the floor and hold on to your ankles. Pull your ankles toward the floor and your knees toward your chest. Relax your neck and shoulders and keep your abdominals strong. Releasing tightness in the buttocks will also help to relax any tension in the hip area.

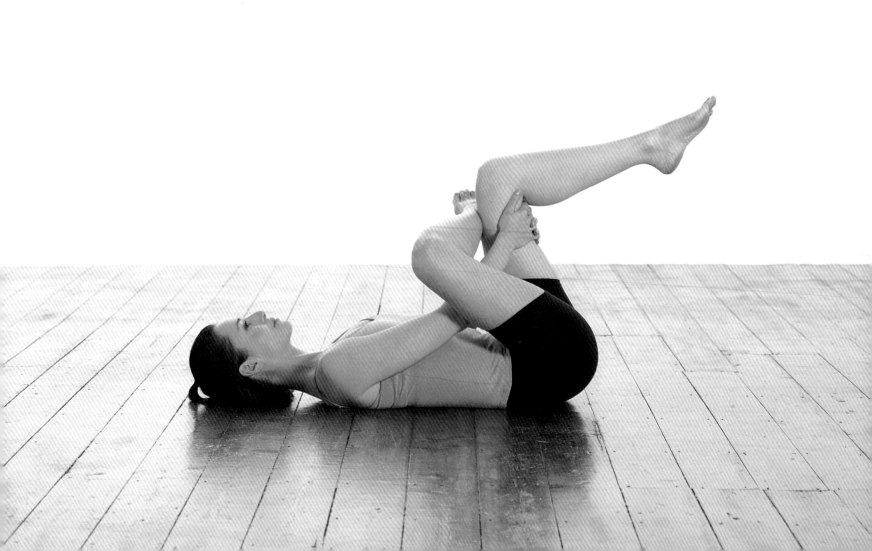

Hamstring stretch

16

 GOOD FOR:
People who do sports,
dancers and anyone
who sits for long
periods of time

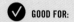 AVOID IF:
You suffer acute low
back pain

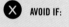 SEE PP.96–7

Lie on your back with both knees bent, feet on the floor hip-width apart. Breathe in as you fold your right knee in toward your chest, lifting your foot off the floor. Clasp your hands behind your right thigh. As you exhale stretch your right leg up toward the ceiling. Keep your tailbone flat on the floor and your abdominals strong. Feel the stretch in the back of the right thigh. Inhale to bend your knee halfway toward your chest, still keeping your tailbone on the floor. Exhale to stretch the leg again. Repeat 5 to 8 times with each leg.

NOTES

This is a very effective stretch if your hamstrings are tight from too much sitting. Make sure you do it gently and be careful not to overstretch your hamstrings. If you are lucky enough to have loose hamstrings, you might like to do the stretch with both legs straight. Keep your tailbone down and be careful not to tilt your pelvis. Your shoulder blades should be relaxed and heavy on the floor. To extend the stretch through the lower leg, pull your toes back toward your body by flexing your ankles. But never force your leg into this position. Alternative hamstring stretches are given in Chapter 3.

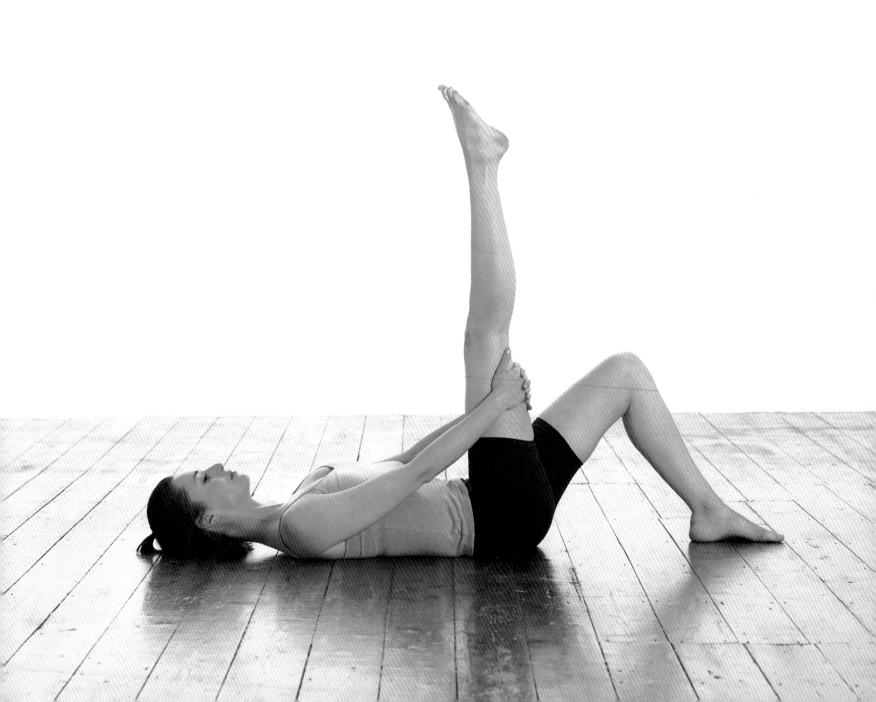

Inner thigh stretch

 GOOD FOR:
Releasing tightness
in the hips, the
inner thighs and
the lower back

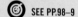 SEE PP.98–9

Sit on the floor with your legs stretched out in front of you. Open them as wide as is comfortable. Try to sit up as high off the "sitting-bones" as possible. Rest your left hand on your left thigh and your right hand on your right thigh. Breathe in. Exhale and lean forward from your hips while keeping your abdominals pulled in. Keep your back long and reach forward from your upper chest down toward the floor. As you breathe in sit up a little, then exhale and reach further forward. Repeat 5 to 8 times.

NOTES

Stretching the inner thighs helps to relieve tension in the hips and the lower spine. This stretch is particularly good for people who ride horses, scooters or motorbikes – actions which require them to "grip" with their inner thighs. Be careful not to bounce while doing this stretch. As you lean forward let your arms guide you by sliding them either along the floor in front of you or down your legs. By flexing your ankles and pulling your toes up you will increase the stretch along the whole inner side of the legs.

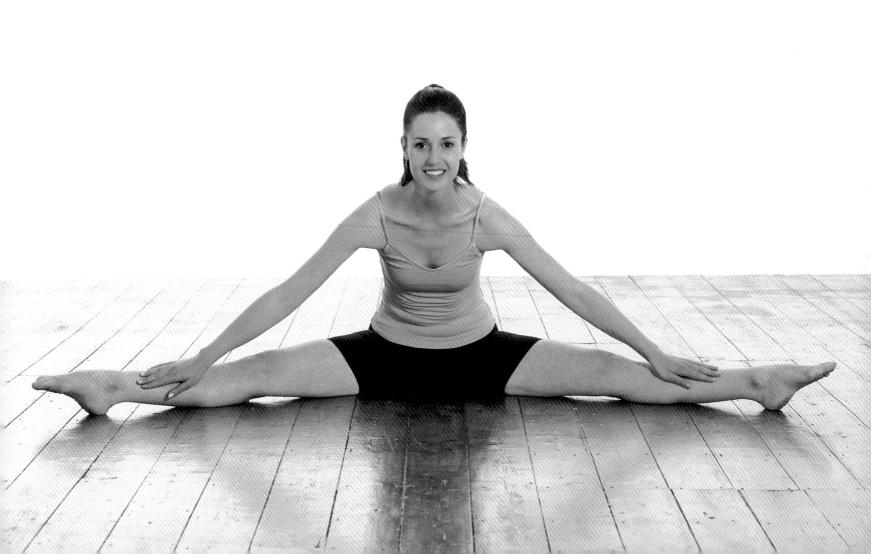

Front of thigh stretch

(18)

✓ **GOOD FOR:**
Cyclists, runners
and people who
do sport in general

✗ **AVOID IF:**
You have knee
replacements

◎ **SEE P.100**

Stand facing the back of a chair or a wall with your left hand holding on for support. Bend your right knee and hold the front of your foot with your right hand. Make sure that your knees are together, your spine is straight and your hips are aligned exactly with your shoulders. Breathe in. As you exhale pull your right leg back slightly, making sure that your abdominals are strong while you maintain the correct spine and hip alignment. You should feel a stretch along the front of your right thigh. Breathe in as you release your knee slightly, then exhale. Repeat 5 to 8 more times.

NOTES

This is an excellent stretch to do after running, cycling and playing sports such as football, which involve a lot of legwork. Be careful not to pull your leg back too far, as this will make your back arch. Keep your abdominals strong throughout to protect your lower back. If you find that this stretch hurts your right shoulder, you could try hooking a towel or band around your foot. The stretch should reach right up to the front of your hip.

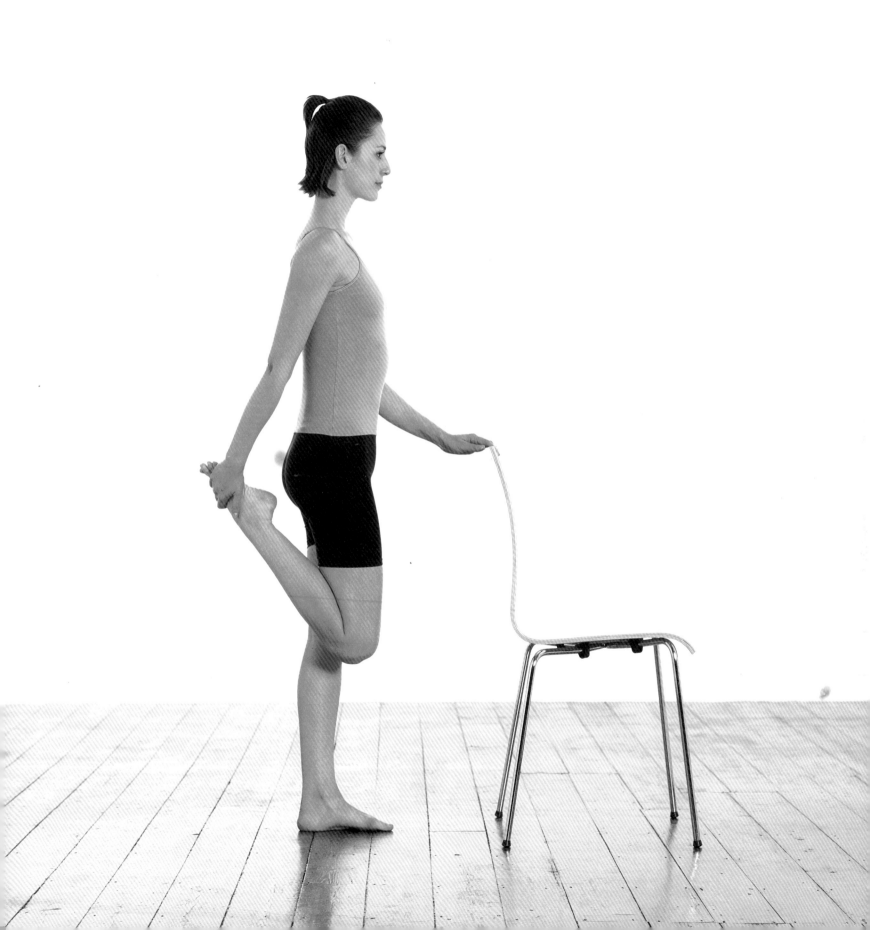

Outer thigh stretch

19

✓ GOOD FOR:
Releasing hip and
lower back tension

◎ SEE P.101

Lie on your back with your feet on the floor hip-width apart, knees bent, and the stretchband in both hands. Bend your right knee in toward your chest and hook the band over your right foot. Stretch your right leg out in front of you and then lift it to a height that feels comfortable for your back. Hold both ends of the band in your left hand. Inhale. Exhale and pull your right leg inward across your body until you feel the stretch on the outside of the thigh. Inhale. Exhale and pull your right leg again to increase the stretch. Now do the stretch with your left leg. Repeat 3 more times with each leg.

NOTES

When you have pulled your leg across your body, you can increase the stretch by flexing your ankle. The outer thigh never gets stretched in everyday activities, so it is important to stretch it to keep it flexible and to release tension in the hip and lower spine. While performing this stretch keep your abdominals strong and relax your shoulders.

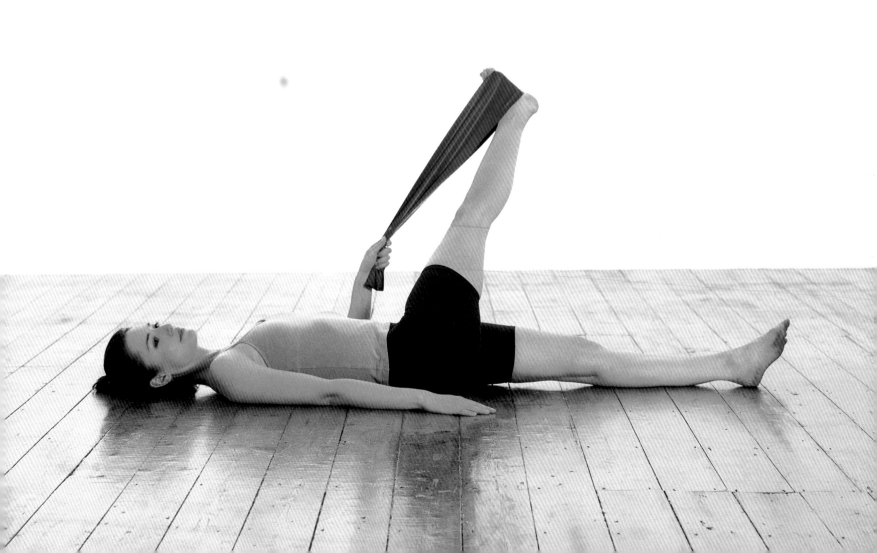

Calf stretch

GOOD FOR:
People who do sport, (especially runners), dancers, and anyone who often wears high-heeled shoes

SEE P.102

Stand facing the back of a chair and rest both hands on it. Bend your left knee and extend your right leg behind you with your right foot flat on the floor. Keeping your body weight forward on your left leg, inhale and reach as far down to the floor as you can with your right heel. Keep your spine in a straight line and maintain strong abdominals. As you exhale, increase the stretch. Then, inhale and relax the stretch a little. Try not to tilt your pelvis – this will make your bottom stick out. Use the chair for support and keep your shoulders relaxed. Repeat the stretch 5 to 8 times on each side.

NOTES

Sometimes we don't realize how stiff our calf muscles are until we stretch them. Walking or standing for long periods in high-heeled shoes can play havoc with our legs. Certain sports make us use our calves a lot – for example running, cycling and football. Dancing, especially ballet, also puts a great deal of strain on the calves. If you want to stretch your deeper calf muscles, slightly bend the leg that is extended behind you, while still trying to keep your heel down. You will feel the difference immediately.

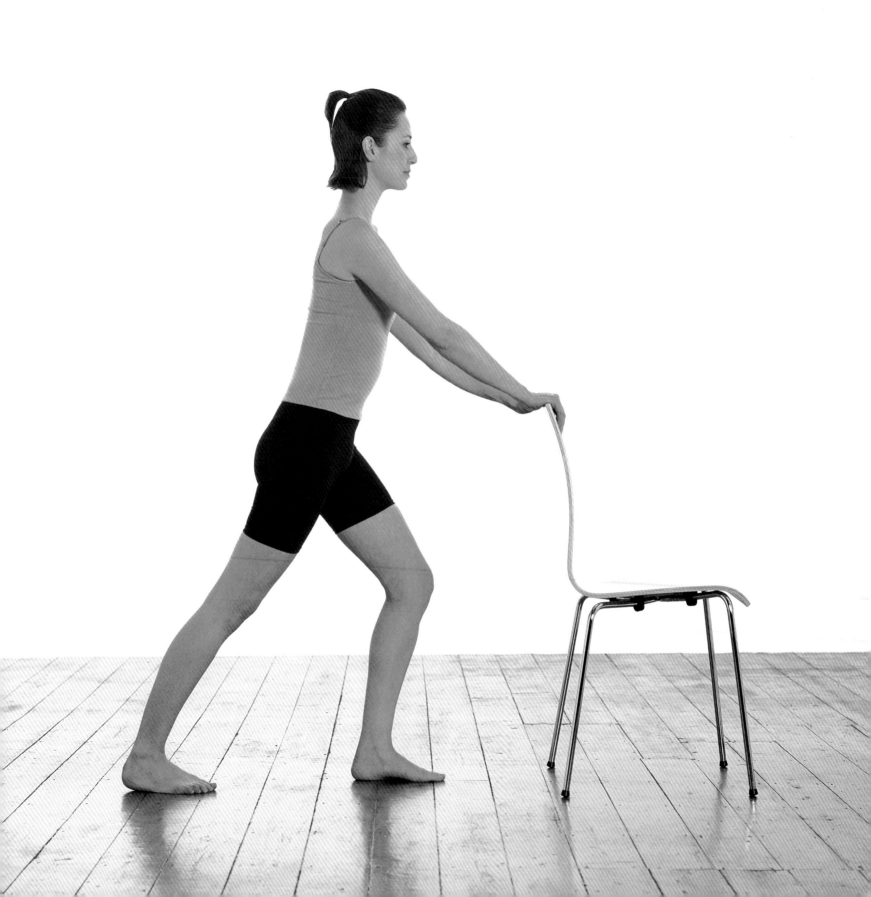

Foot and ankle stretch

GOOD FOR:

Strengthening
weak feet, calves
and ankles

SEE P.103

You may like to try this stretch holding on to a chair for support at first. Stand with your feet hip-width apart. Keep your back long and your abdominals strong. As you inhale, shift your weight forward on to the balls of your feet and rise up on your toes. In this position you will feel your calf muscles tighten and the front of your feet and ankles stretch. Breathe out as you lower your heels in a controlled way. Repeat 8 to 10 times.

NOTES

As well as stretching the feet and the ankles, this exercise is good for practising balance. As you rise up on your toes, imagine that you are being pulled up by a hair on the top of your head. Visualize a straight line running down the centre of your body down to the floor between each heel. Make sure you keep your weight over the centre of each foot. Keep your ankles straight so that they don't twist or roll outward. You may like to place a tennis ball between your ankles to help you maintain the correct alignment. With practice you will be able to do this stretch without a chair for support.

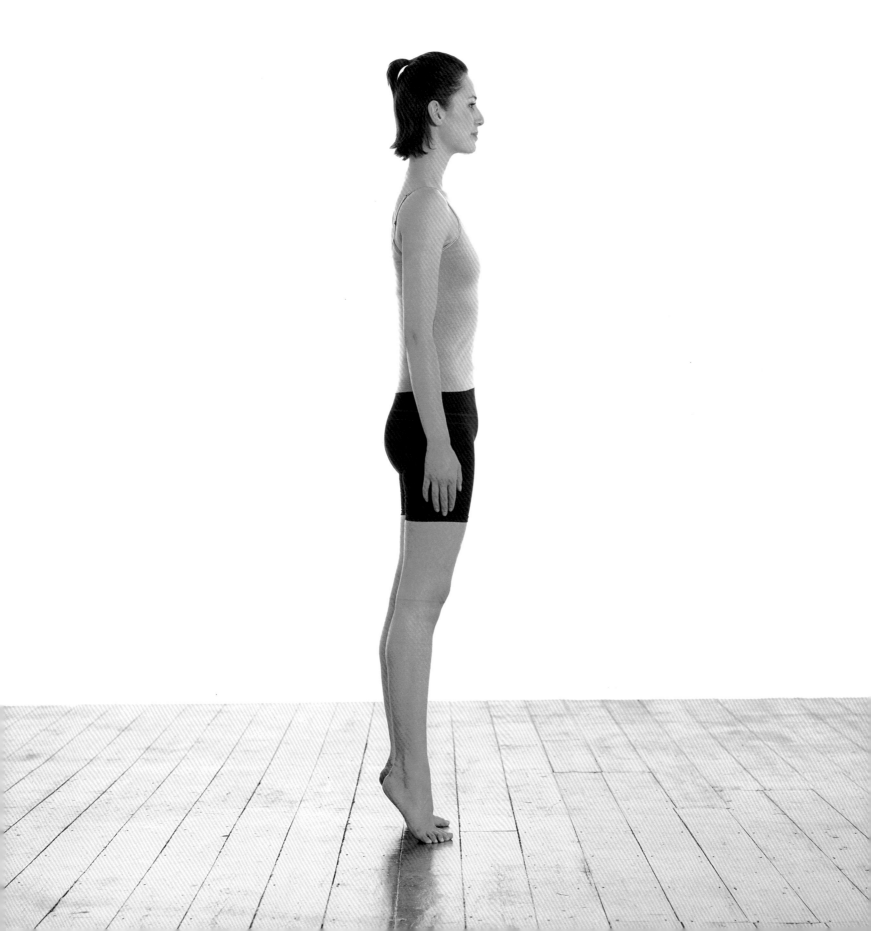

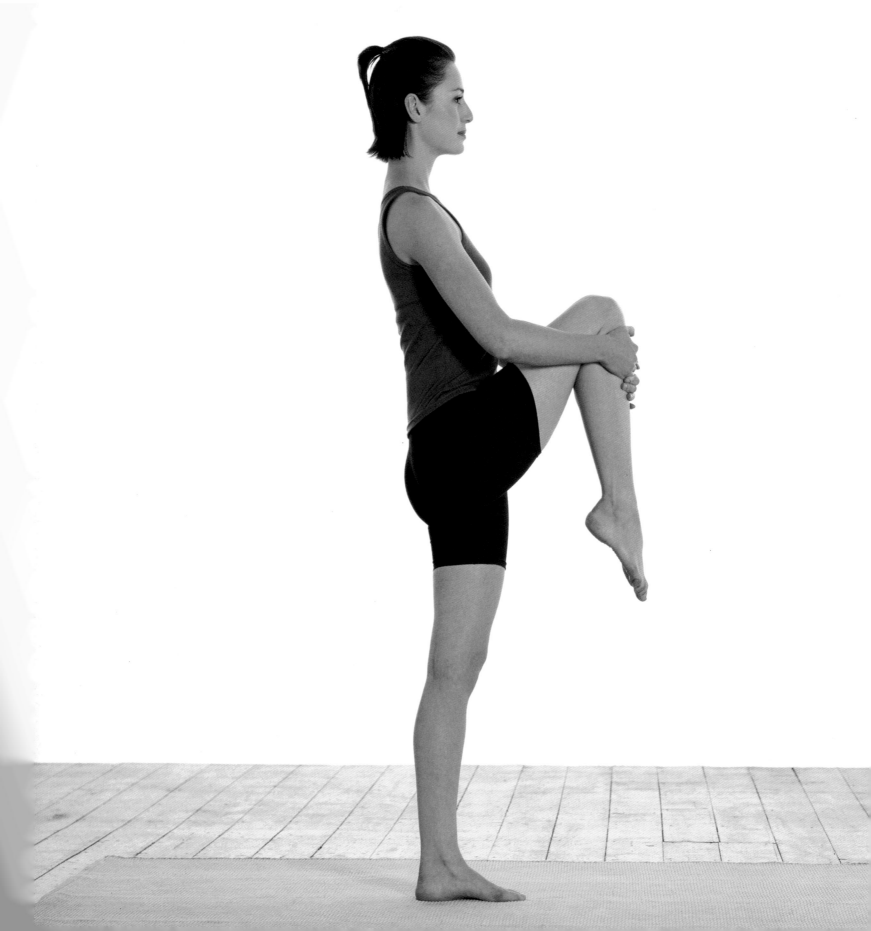

CHAPTER 3:
Easy Solutions

We each have our own physical identity. Changes in circumstances can affect the way we feel from day to day, causing stress which can manifest itself physically in the form of common ailments, such as tension headaches, backache and shoulder strain. It is therefore important to take into account how you feel when you start a stretching session, and to adapt the exercises to meet your physical requirements that day. Whichever stretches you select, aim to achieve a balance of strength, serenity, poise and precision.

If you have been finding any of the stretches in Chapter 2 at all difficult, this chapter will help you by suggesting easier solutions and alternative positions.

How to modify a stretch

If you feel a bit daunted by some of the stretches shown in Chapter 2, don't worry! Remember that these are target positions and it is unlikely that you will be able to achieve them when you begin. But, as your body becomes more relaxed and flexible, it will also become easier to perform the stretches.

In the meantime I have suggested a series of easier or alternative stretches. Take time to try out the various options and choose the position that feels best for you. Remember to modify the stretch according to your needs. For example, if you have spent a weekend gardening and you wake up on Monday morning with backache, you should avoid stretching your spine too much and select one of the easier back stretches, such as the modified Kneeling Back Stretch (see p.89).

THE MIND—BODY CONNECTION

By focusing on your body as you stretch, you will become more aware of the areas that are tight and need to be more supple. Try to work out why a particular area is tense. Could it be because of the way you habitually sit, stand, drive or sleep? When you have pinpointed the reason for the tension or stiffness, you will find it is much easier to rectify the problem. Also, the way you think about your body influences the way in which it functions. So, once you start to think positively about stretching you will find that you progress faster and easier.

MOVING OR NON-MOVING

A stretch can also be made easier by practising it statically or dynamically. Static or non-moving stretching is when you reach the target position and stay in it for a few breaths. An example of a static stretch would be the second modified position of the Spine Twist (see p.85). Once you have reached the correct position you remain there for a few breaths before returning to the starting position.

Dynamic or moving stretching is when you reach the target position and then gradually stretch a little further. You are in control of the movement so that you can gently push yourself to the limits of your ability. An example of a dynamic stretch would be the first modified position of the Hamstring Stretch (see p.96). Gently increase the stretch by pulling the stretchband further back. In this way you can control the limit to which you try to stretch your leg.

In addition to the static and dynamic methods of stretching, there is another type: passive stretching. This involves relaxing into the stretch as much as possible in order to release deep tension. An example of a completely passive stretch would be the second Inner Thigh modified position (see p.99). As you relax into the stretch, gravity is doing the work by allowing the hips and inner thighs to be stretched passively.

Creating an easy routine

When planning a stretching routine, it is important to consider the practicalities. If you are practising at home, you need to use a quiet room that has enough space for you to lie down comfortably on the floor and stretch out your whole body. If there is a telephone in that room, switch the ring to a low volume or set the answerphone. Play some music that inspires you to stretch and energize your body. Classical or relaxation music is most appropriate, as anything with a fast rhythm might encourage you to bounce or perform the movements too jerkily.

Use an exercise mat or towel to lie on, and if necessary, support your head on a cushion or a book. Ideally, when lying on your back, your head should be straight and in line with your neck and spine. People with abnormal or exaggerated curvature of the spine often have a slight tilt of the head when lying flat. If your hair is long, tie it back at the nape of your neck or high up on your head.

It is a good idea to use a large mirror to monitor yourself as you do the exercises, so that you can check your postural alignment. (If your alignment is incorrect you will not benefit as much from the stretches and you could put additional strain on your body.)

It is wise to do only the standing and sitting stretches if you have a cold or blocked sinuses, as lying down can increase head and nasal congestion. And, if time is limited, just choose a few of the stretches. It is better to do some rather than none at all. Make your stretching routine fit in with your lifestyle. For example, if you work all day, do your stretching first thing in the morning, or in the evening when you come home.

WHICH PART DO I STRETCH FIRST?

There is no set rule concerning which area of the body should be stretched first. In this book I have started from the top of the body and worked down to the feet. When you stretch you are generally exercising more than one muscle at a time. Although you may be trying to work one particular muscle or muscle group, there are usually supporting muscles also involved. In Chapter 2, I have deliberately put the lower back, buttock and hip stretches before the hamstrings stretch, because by stretching the areas that support your hamstrings first, you relax them, and by so doing make your hamstrings easier to stretch.

If you have injured a particular part of your body and have been advised not to move it, you can still keep stretching the other areas. For example, if you have broken or sprained your ankle badly and you need crutches, keep stretching your neck and shoulders, as using crutches can strain your upper body.

Above all, bear in mind that stretching is all about extending yourself and stretching your boundaries as well as your muscles.

Head tilt

SOLUTION

Problems with this stretch are usually caused by having a stiff neck. This could be because of the way you work or sleep; or because you have been sitting in a draught. (Although a stretchband is used in the target position, you do not need one for this modified stretch.)

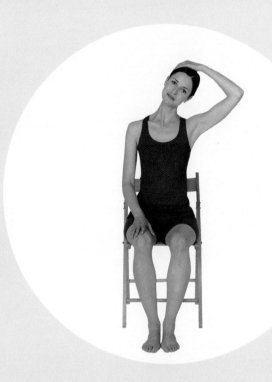

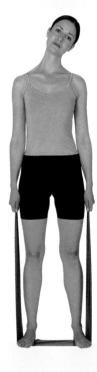

target
position

SEE PP.30–31

❌ PROBLEM: The stretch pulls too much on my neck and my back tends to arch.

✔ SOLUTION: Sit on a chair and keep your spine straight. Then, pull your head gently to one side with your hand.

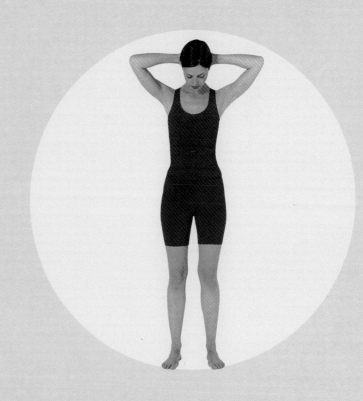

Head nod

SOLUTION

Problems with stretching the neck are usually related to habitual bad posture, such as sitting with your head forward when using a computer, or sleeping on too many pillows. (Although a stretchband is used in the target position, you do not need one for this modified stretch.)

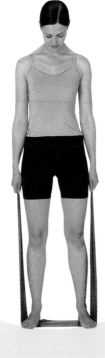

target
position

SEE PP.32–3

❌ PROBLEM: **The stretch pulls too much in my shoulders.**

✅ SOLUTION: **Clasp your hands at the back of your head and gently pull it forward. Don't overstretch. Try to keep your elbows slightly open and your shoulders relaxed.**

Shoulder release
SOLUTIONS

Shoulder tension is usually caused by weakness in the neck, upper back or arms. Driving and carrying heavy objects can often make the shoulders tighten. (Although a stretchband is used in the target position, you do not need one for the modified stretches.)

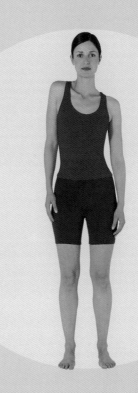

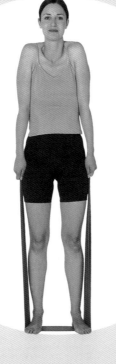

target position

SEE PP.34–5

❌ PROBLEM: **My shoulders ache when I use the stretchband.**

✔️ SOLUTION: **Simply do the same stretch without the band and make it easier by exercising one shoulder at a time.**

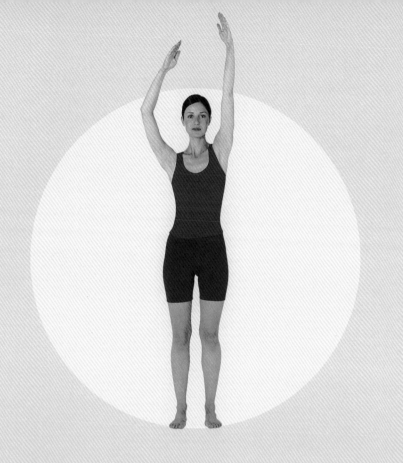

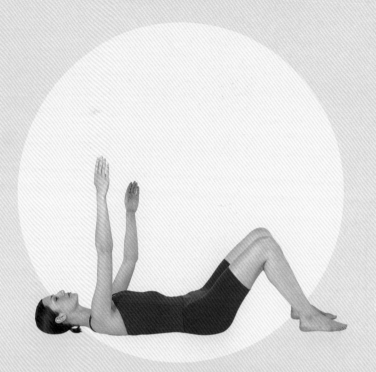

ⓧ PROBLEM: I am only feeling the stretch at the top of my shoulders.

✓ SOLUTION: Try lifting both arms up and stretching one arm at a time. This will target the front and sides of the shoulders more.

ⓧ PROBLEM: I am unable to maintain the correct spinal alignment. I find myself arching my back automatically.

✓ SOLUTION: Lie on your back with both knees bent, your spine relaxed. Reach up, one arm at a time, to stretch your shoulders. In between stretches, relax the arm and shoulder you've just stretched back down.

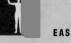

Upper chest and shoulder stretch

SOLUTIONS

Tightness in the shoulders and the chest is common because many of us sit incorrectly — in the correct posture, our shoulders align with our hips. (Although a stretchband is used in the target position, you do not need one for this modified stretch.)

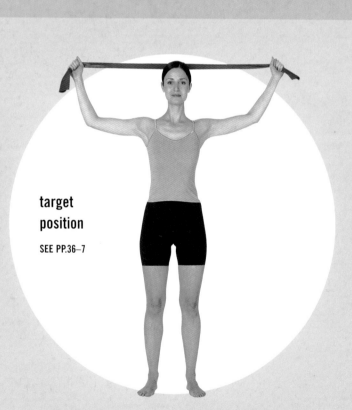

target position

SEE PP.36–7

❌ PROBLEM: **When I lift up my arms, my back wants to arch and my head leans forward.**

✓ SOLUTION: **Lie on your right side, with your knees bent, arms outstretched and spine straight. As you inhale lift your right arm and turn your head toward it. Exhale and stretch this arm, keeping the elbow soft. Don't move your hips. Inhale and bring the arm back, then exhale. Repeat five times with each arm.**

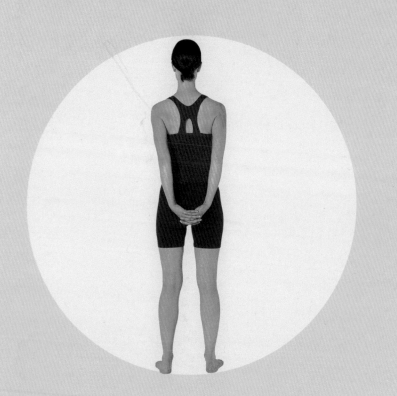

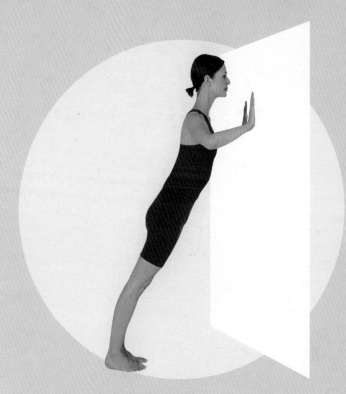

❌ PROBLEM: **My arms hurt when I lift them up above my head.**

✅ SOLUTION: **Clasp your hands behind your back and stretch your arms as much as you can. Be careful not to lock your elbows and make sure that your shoulders stay down.**

❌ PROBLEM: **I am unable to pull the band behind my head and shoulders.**

✅ SOLUTION: **Stand in a doorway with your arms bent, hands a bit higher than shoulder height, resting on the doorframe. Inhale. As you exhale lean forward through the door, keeping your back straight and your abdominals strong.**

Upper arm and shoulder pull

SOLUTIONS

You may find this stretch uncomfortable at first if your wrists and arms are tight from using a computer. Start with one of the modified stretches and when this feels comfortable, progress to the target position.

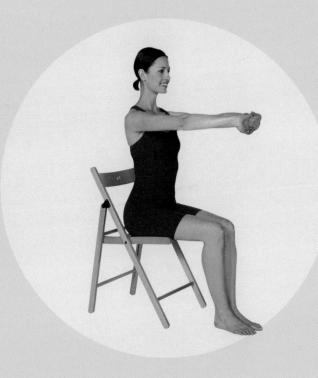

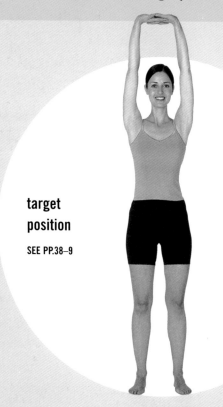

target position

SEE PP.38–9

❌ PROBLEM: **I find it difficult doing this stretch with my arms lifted.**

✅ SOLUTION: **Sit in a chair with your back straight and your arms outstretched at shoulder height. Clasp your hands, breathe out and stretch forward with your palms.**

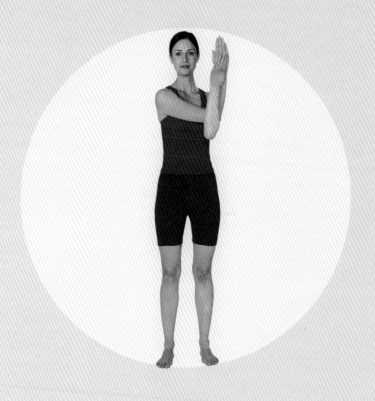

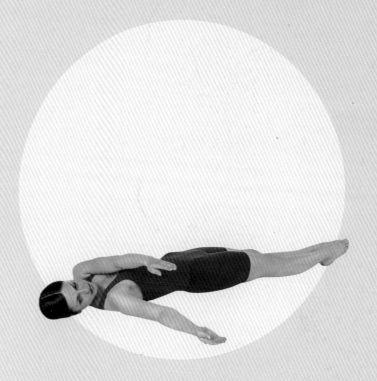

⊗ PROBLEM: **I find it difficult to feel the stretch in my shoulders.**

✓ SOLUTION: **Either stand or sit and cross your arms at the elbows, your arms in front of your chest. Inhale. As you exhale pull both arms across your body. If your right arm is on the outside, pull your arms to the right; if your left arm is on the outside, pull your arms to the left. Repeat five times with each arm.**

⊗ PROBLEM: **I find it difficult to stand with my spine straight and my arms up – my back arches.**

✓ SOLUTION: **Lie on the floor on your back, with either bent or straight legs, your arms out to the side at 90°. Inhale. As you exhale bring your left arm across your body and reach toward your right arm. Repeat, this time bringing your right arm across your body.**

Spine twist
SOLUTIONS

Any of the spine-twist stretches are good to do daily. Make sure that you keep your abdominals strong whichever stretch you choose. If you are finding this stretch difficult to do, the cause might be tight hips or buttocks, or your lower back might have restricted mobility.

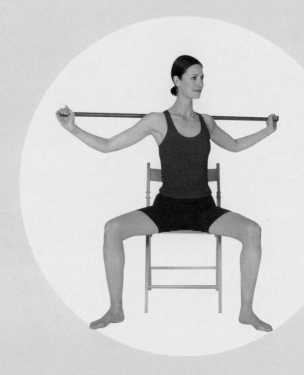

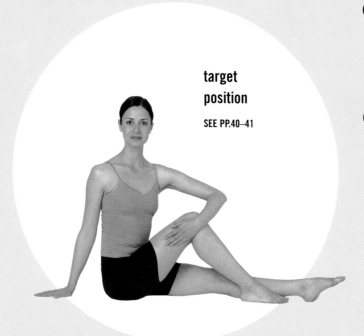

target
position

SEE PP.40–41

❌ PROBLEM: **I find it difficult to open out my shoulders and keep my back straight.**

✓ SOLUTION: **Sit on a chair with your back straight. Place a pole or a broom handle across the back of your shoulders and hold it with your palms facing forward. Breathe in. Exhale and twist your spine to the left, keeping your hips still. The pole will help you to keep your shoulders open.**

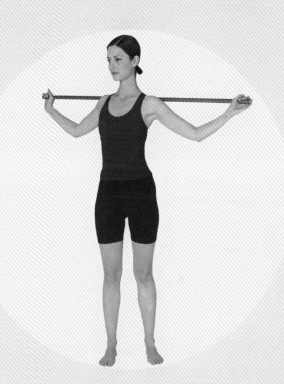

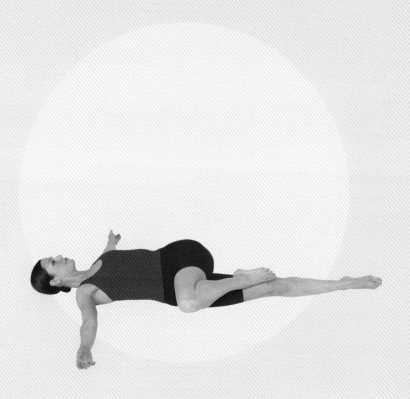

X PROBLEM: **I find it difficult to sit in the target position.**

✔ SOLUTION: **Lie on your back, both legs straight, arms extended out at 90° to the side. Inhale and bend your left leg up toward you. Exhale as you pull your left leg over to your right side, so that your spine twists. Look up or turn your head slightly to your right. Relax both shoulders and rest them firmly on the floor.**

X PROBLEM: **I am unable to twist my spine very much.**

✔ SOLUTION: **Begin by rotating your spine only slightly. Stand holding a pole across the back of your shoulders. Try to keep your hips still. Exhale as you gently twist your spine to the left.**

Spine stretch forward

SOLUTION

This stretch can be difficult if your hamstrings are tight, your lower back is stiff or your abdominals are weak. By taking the weight off your legs and lower spine you should find it easier to use your abdominals.

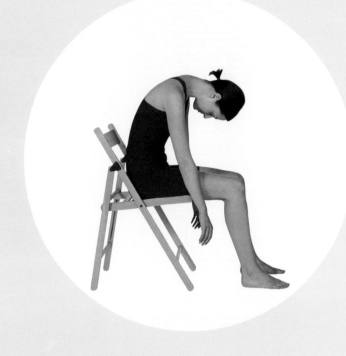

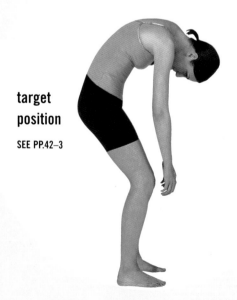

target position

SEE PP.42–3

❌ PROBLEM: **The back of my thighs and lower back feel tight.**

✅ SOLUTION: **Do the same stretch sitting in a chair to take the strain off your legs. As you breathe out nod your head and allow its weight to roll your spine slowly forward so that your head drops down between your knees. Breathe in while you are in this position and breathe out again as you roll your spine back up.**

Spine stretch back
SOLUTION

This stretch can feel awkward if your abdominals are not strong enough to support the position of your spine, or if you find it hard to keep your shoulders pulled down. Try the following alternative stretch, but remember to pull in your abdominals.

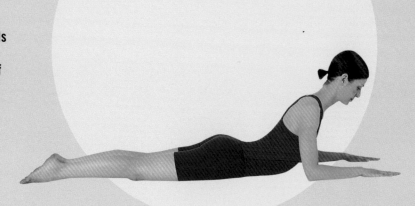

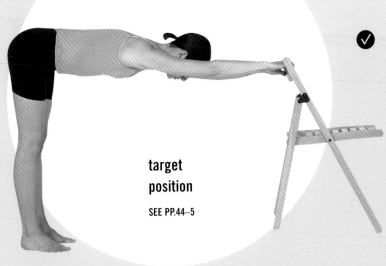

target
position

SEE PP.44–5

❌ PROBLEM: I find it hard to lean forward without my back curving.

✅ SOLUTION: Lie on your front with your arms bent, your hands slightly forward from your shoulders. Breathe in. As you exhale pull in your abdominals, draw your shoulders down into your back and lift your upper body away from the floor. Don't lift your head too much. Your neck should remain long.

Chest curl

SOLUTION

This movement can be difficult to perform if your abdominal muscles are weak. You may feel tension at the back of your neck or in the front of your hips and thighs. Try to let your head rest back in your hands when you lift it, so that you do not overstretch or strain your neck.

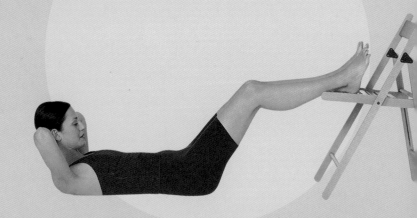

target position

SEE PP.46–7

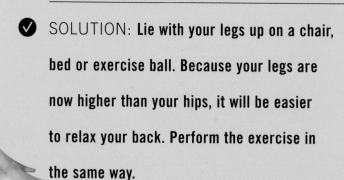

❌ PROBLEM: **I am unable to keep my back relaxed and flat on the floor and my pelvis moves when I curl up.**

✔ SOLUTION: **Lie with your legs up on a chair, bed or exercise ball. Because your legs are now higher than your hips, it will be easier to relax your back. Perform the exercise in the same way.**

Kneeling back stretch

SOLUTION

This stretch is often difficult if you have a stiff lower back. To make it easier try placing cushions under your forehead and your buttocks. If you have any knee problems, try the alternative stretch instead.

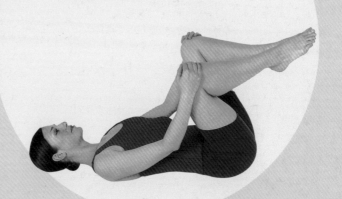

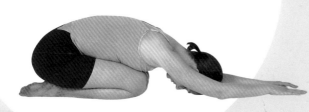

target
position

SEE PP.48–9

 PROBLEM: I am unable to get my head and tailbone down toward the floor and the fronts of my feet are uncomfortable.

 SOLUTION: **Lie on your back and bend both knees toward your chest. Keep your feet together and your knees slightly wider than hip-width apart. As you breathe in place your hands on your knees and then as you exhale pull your knees toward your chest and shoulders.**

Waist stretch
SOLUTIONS

Bending to the side can be problematic if you have any tightness in your lower back or hips. Using the stretchband will give you the maximum stretch, but if you do not have one or prefer to stretch without a band, try the second or third modified stretches.

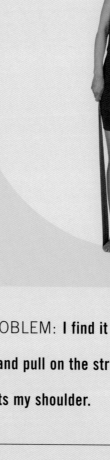

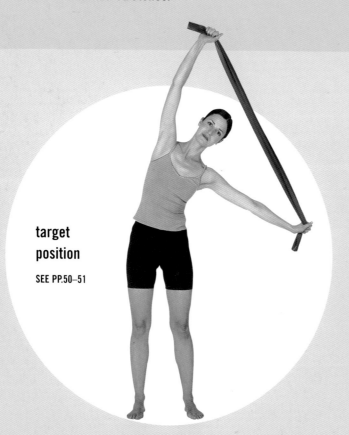

target position

SEE PP.50–51

❌ PROBLEM: **I find it difficult to hold my arms up and pull on the stretchband as this action hurts my shoulder.**

✔ SOLUTION: **Do the same exercise, but this time standing on the band. You will still benefit from stretching against resistance, but holding your arms down by your sides will be easier on your shoulders. Keep your hips still as you bend.**

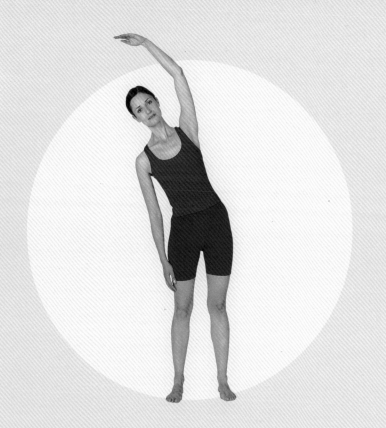

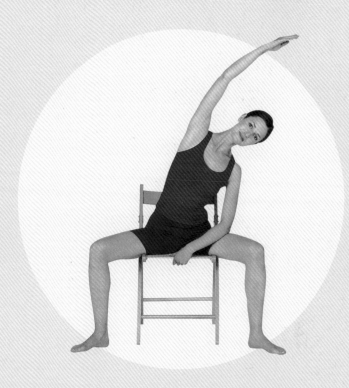

❌ PROBLEM: **I find it hard to keep my shoulders down when I lift my arms above my head.**

✔ SOLUTION: **Try lifting one arm at a time without the band. Breathe in as you raise your left arm. Exhale as you stretch over to your right side, reaching across with your arm and your hand. Repeat on the other side.**

❌ PROBLEM: **I feel tense in my lower back and I find it difficult to keep my hips still when I bend.**

✔ SOLUTION: **Sit on a chair to do the same stretch. Hold on to the front of the seat with your left hand as you stretch over to the left with your right arm.**

Front of hip stretch
SOLUTION

This stretch is fairly difficult, as it requires both balance and strength to hold the position. To begin with you could try the alternative using the chair. You could then try the target position with both hands on the floor instead of on your thigh.

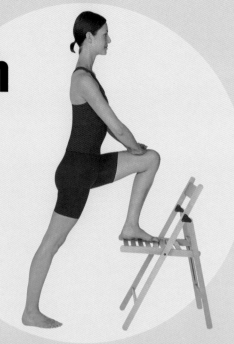

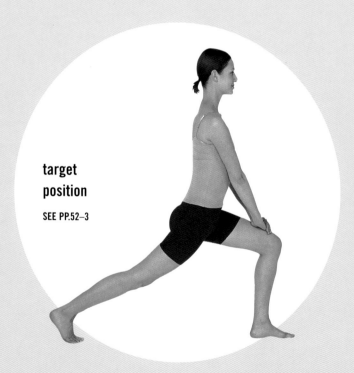

target position

SEE PP.52–3

⊗ PROBLEM: **I find it very difficult to keep my spine straight without feeling discomfort in my lower back.**

✓ SOLUTION: **Use a chair to support one leg. Place your left leg on the chair and bend your knee. Rest your hands on your thigh. Stand with your back straight. Inhale. Exhale and lean forward keeping your back straight and your pelvis neutral.**

Side of hip stretch

SOLUTION

This is a straightforward stretch. However, it is sometimes difficult to maintain your spine in the correct position and to feel the stretch in the right areas: at the side of the hip, in the buttock and the lower back. Ensure that you don't roll too far as this will make you arch your back.

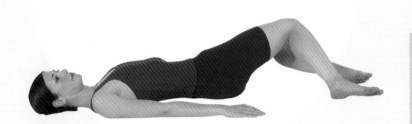

target
position

SEE PP.54–5

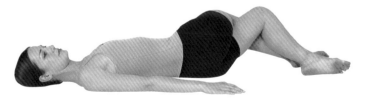

✗ PROBLEM: I find it awkward to keep my legs crossed and to roll my hips at the same time, without putting pressure on my lower back.

✓ SOLUTION: Do the same exercise with your legs uncrossed, about hip-width apart. You may find it more comfortable if you place a cushion between your knees.

Buttock stretch

SOLUTIONS

This stretch can feel rather awkward at first. However, once you master the movement you will feel the stretch in your deep buttock muscles and also around your hip. This stretch is particularly good if you have sciatica. Here, I have suggested three alternative stretches.

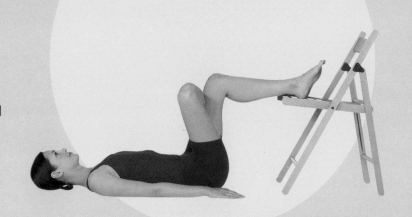

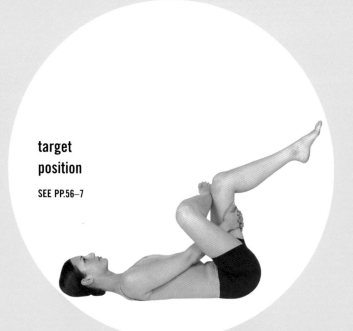

target
position

SEE PP.56–7

❌ PROBLEM: **I find it difficult to reach the back of my thigh and clasp my hands without my shoulders tensing.**

✔ SOLUTION: **Use a chair. Bend your left leg and rest your left foot on the chair. Bend your right knee and place your ankle across the front of your left knee. Relax and breathe deeply in this position. The closer you are to the chair, the more you will be stretching.**

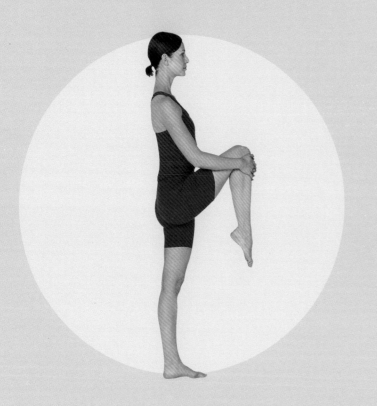

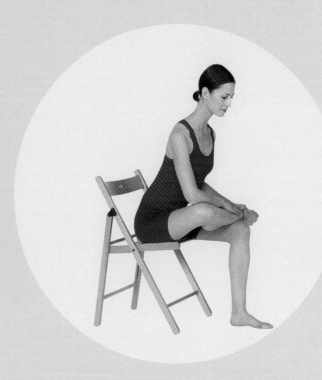

✕ PROBLEM: I find it uncomfortable to open my knee outward because my hips are so tight.

✕ PROBLEM: I would like to stretch my buttocks and hips without having to lie on the floor

✓ SOLUTION: You could try the target position without opening your right knee. Or try standing on your left leg and hug your right knee to your chest. This is also good for your balance. Remember to keep your back straight and your abdominals strong.

✓ SOLUTION: Sit with your right leg bent across the other, your knee open, your right elbow resting on your leg. Breathe in. As you exhale lean forward keeping your back as straight as possible. Let your elbow gently push your right knee down.

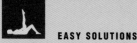

Hamstring stretch

SOLUTIONS

This can be a difficult stretch unless you are lucky enough to have loose hamstrings and good flexibility in your hips. For this reason I have shown three alternative solutions. Approach this stretch gently, as it is easy to injure the hamstring muscles.

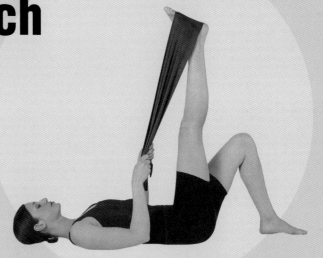

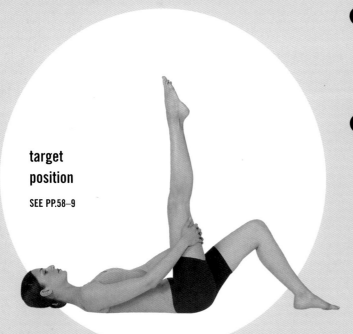

target position

SEE PP.58–9

✕ PROBLEM: **I cannot reach my leg to pull it back toward my chest.**

✓ SOLUTION: **Do the same stretch using the stretchband. The resistance will allow you to rest your arms, and relax your shoulders while you still get a good stretch. If you feel your back arching, bend your left leg more.**

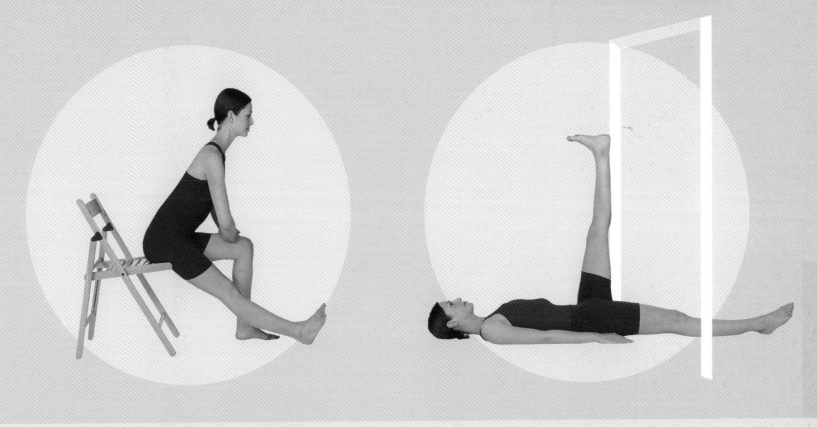

✗ PROBLEM: I find it difficult to maintain a straight back and keep my tailbone down when I pull my leg back.

✓ SOLUTION: Sit on a chair with your right leg straight out in front of you. Breathe in. As you exhale hinge forward from the hips and flex your right ankle so that your toes are pulling upward. It is important to keep your back straight as you lean forward. Rest your arms on your left thigh.

✗ PROBLEM: I find this places a strain on my shoulders as my arms are quite short.

✓ SOLUTION: Lie on the floor with your right leg through a doorway. Lift your left leg and rest it against the doorframe. Let your arms relax by your sides. If you feel your lower back arching, bend your right leg.

Inner thigh stretch
SOLUTIONS

This stretch can be difficult if you have tight hips and inner thighs. Sitting cross-legged for long periods of time can create a lot of tension in these areas. Try one of the three alternative stretches I suggest here until your hips start to feel looser.

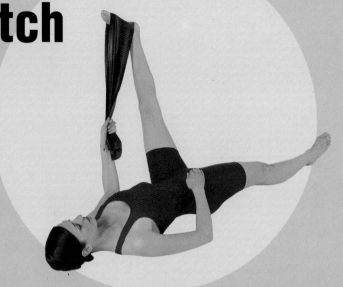

target position

SEE PP.60–61

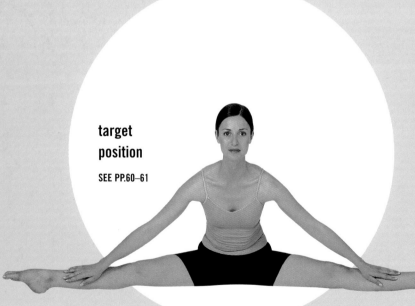

⊗ PROBLEM: I feel imbalanced in this position as one side seems tighter than the other.

✓ SOLUTION: Lie on your back with the stretchband around your left foot, your left leg elevated. Hold both ends of the band with your left hand and place your right hand on your right hip to stabilize it. Breathe in. As you exhale gently pull your left leg outward from the hip, keeping your right hip still.

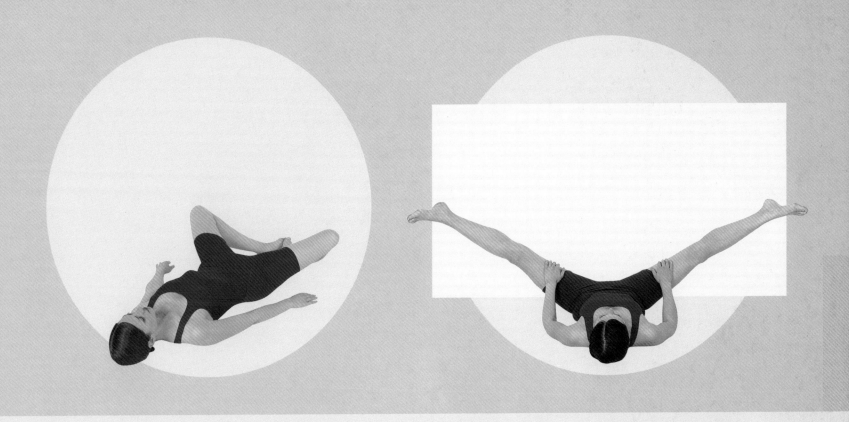

X PROBLEM: **I feel too much of a pull in my inner thighs and hamstrings as I lean forward.**

✓ SOLUTION: **Try the same stretch without leaning forward, keeping your feet relaxed. Or, you could lie on your back with your knees bent and the soles of your feet together. This is a good, passive stretch to open the hips and stretch the inner thighs. You might like to place a cushion under each thigh for comfort.**

X PROBLEM: **I find it difficult to keep my back straight when sitting with my legs outstretched.**

✓ SOLUTION: **Sit in front of a wall with both your knees bent. Lie on your back, open out your legs and rest them against the wall. You will find that your back relaxes and your legs gradually open out further as you stretch your inner thighs.**

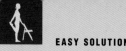
Front of thigh stretch
SOLUTION

Many people are advised to perform this stretch after running and cycling, as it releases tension from the quadriceps muscles. I suggest using a chair or a wall for support, as it can be quite difficult to balance on one leg and maintain the correct alignment between the spine and pelvis.

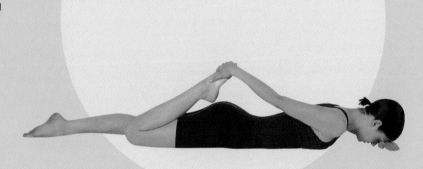

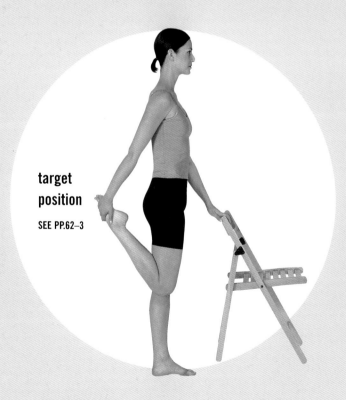

target
position

SEE PP.62–3

❌ PROBLEM: I find it difficult to keep my back straight while keeping my spine and pelvis in alignment.

✓ SOLUTION: Lie on your stomach on the floor, your head resting on your left hand. Bend your right knee and hold your right foot with your right hand. Exhale as you pull your foot toward your buttock. If you can't reach your foot, hook the stretchband around it.

Outer thigh stretch
SOLUTION

This part of the body is sometimes neglected in stretching and strengthening exercises. In fact, the outer and inner thighs a play a vital part in keeping the hip and knee joints stable. (Although a stretchband is used in the target position, you do not need one for this modified stretch.)

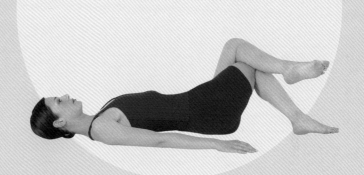

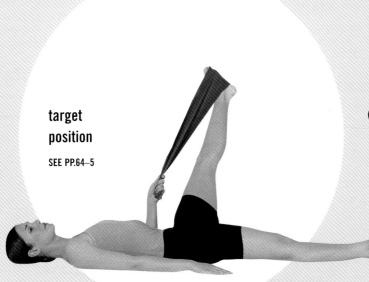

target position

SEE PP.64–5

❌ PROBLEM: Because my hamstrings are tight, I find it difficult to keep my leg straight and pull it to one side.

✔ SOLUTION: Lie on your back with your left leg crossed over your right leg. Roll your hips to your left, using your left leg as a lever to pull the right leg into the stretch.

Calf stretch

SOLUTION

If you walk, run, play sport or dance regularly, you need to stretch your calves every day. If you don't stretch your calf muscles regularly you might become susceptible to cramps. However, take care not to overstretch either, otherwise you could strain the Achilles tendons at the back of your ankles.

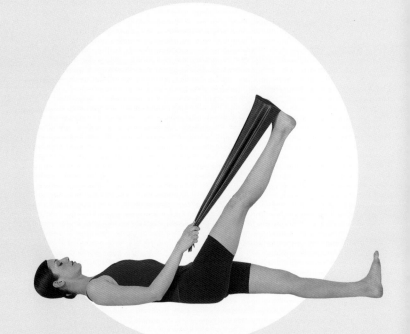

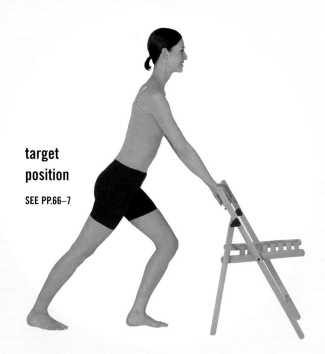

target position

SEE PP.66–7

✗ PROBLEM: When I lean forward I can't keep my back straight and my pelvis aligned, or put my foot flat on the floor.

✓ SOLUTION: Try combining the calf and hamstring stretches, using the stretchband. Lie on your back with your right leg elevated and the band around the right foot. Pull your toes back toward you – you will feel the stretch from the heel right up through the calf.

CALF STRETCH • FOOT AND ANKLE STRETCH

Foot and ankle stretch

SOLUTION

Although this stretch appears to be quite easy, it is actually quite difficult to keep your feet correctly aligned. Keep your body weight distributed evenly on both feet, in particular on your big toes, as these are the strongest toes.

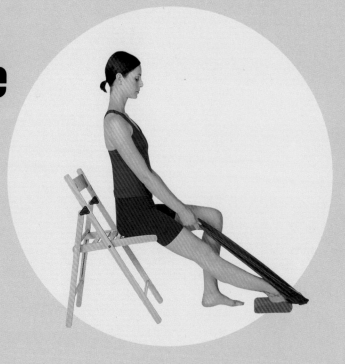

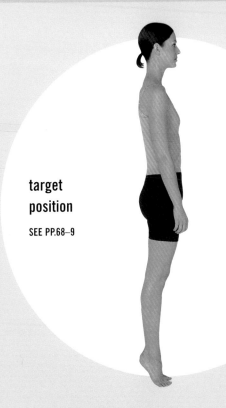

target
position

SEE PP.68–9

❌ PROBLEM: **I feel the stretch at the front of my ankle and in my instep, but not in my toes because I can't rise up very high on them.**

✔ SOLUTION: **Sit on a chair. Stretch out your right leg and rest the foot on a cushion. Wrap the stretchband around all the toes of your right foot. Point your toes downward, then lift them up again. Do this several times. Repeat with the stretchband around your other foot.**

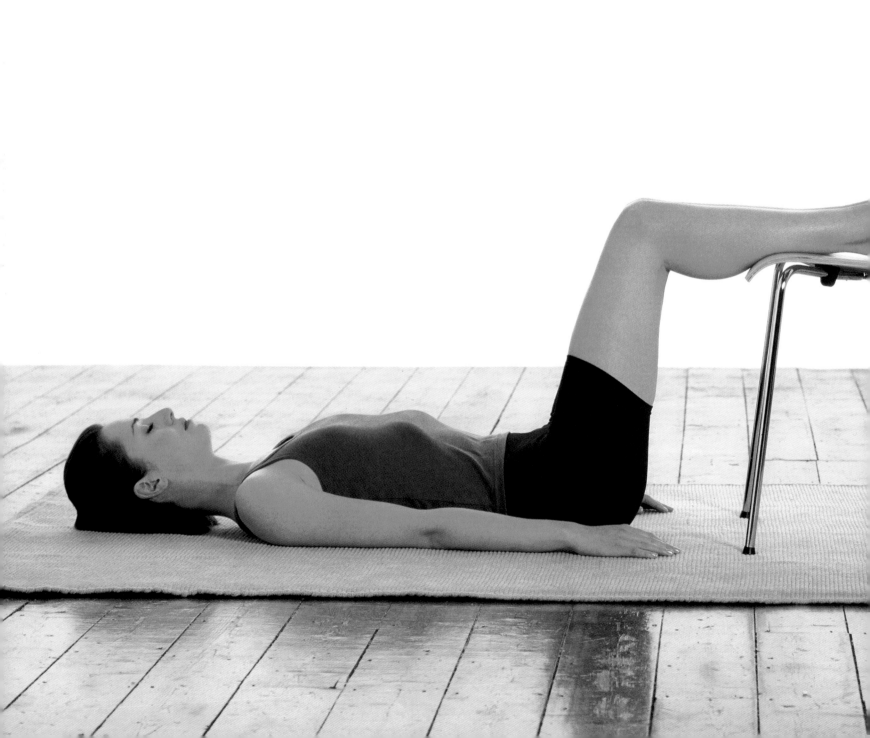

CHAPTER 4:
Easy Relaxation

Relaxing at the end of your stretching session will give both your body and your mind a chance to absorb the benefits of your practice. However, if you want to optimize your health you need to incorporate some form of daily relaxation into your life to help you wind down after a busy day. Many people feel that watching television or reading is relaxing, but this is untrue – the eyes and the brain have to work hard during these activities. True relaxation does not require any equipment and it costs nothing except time and motivation.

This chapter takes you through a series of relaxation, breathing and meditation exercises. If you practise them regularly, you will find that you are better equipped to deal with all types of stress.

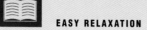

Progressive muscular relaxation

Progressive muscular relaxation relieves tension by relaxing muscle groups individually. As the name suggests the idea is to work progressively through the body, systematically flexing and relaxing muscle groups.

In all, the following relaxation exercise should take around 10 to 15 minutes to perform. It will make you aware of the areas in which you hold the most tension, and when combined with the breathing exercises, it will promote deep relaxation.

Lie with your knees bent, feet hip-width apart. Relax your arms by your sides slightly away from your body, and rest the backs of your hands on the floor. Be aware of your surroundings, then close your eyes. Let your eyes feel heavy beneath your eyelids. Relax your jaw so that your teeth separate slightly and smile a little to relax your face. Swallow to relax the throat and front of neck. Imagine that you are lying in sand and your whole body is sinking into it. The backs of your shoulders and your ribs feel heavy, and your hips also feel weighted down in the imaginary sand. Stretch and part your legs and relax them and your feet completely. Now focus on your breathing, and observe how easily it enters and leaves your body.

If you find it comfortable, move your arms up alongside your head. If not, leave them at your sides. Stretch your fingers and toes as much as you can, as if you are being pulled

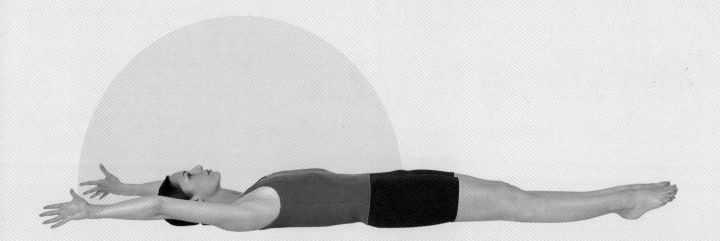

from both ends of the body. Feel the tension in the muscles of your feet and hands. Hold this stretch for a count of ten and then relax. Now stretch your calves and knees, elbows and forearms. Tighten all these muscles and notice how that tightness feels, while at the same time trying to keep your fingers and toes relaxed. You are aiming to isolate one area of the body from another. After a count of ten, relax your calves, knees, elbows and forearms. Now tighten your thighs and buttocks, and relax them after you have counted to ten. Moving on to the abdominal area, try to engage your pelvic floor muscles at the same time as drawing your abdominal muscles down toward the floor without moving your pelvis, so that your stomach becomes flatter. Moving up to the shoulders, slide them up toward your ears so that your neck disappears. Finally, feel the tension in the tops of your shoulders and then relax and slide them down toward your rib-cage so that your neck becomes long again and your shoulders become heavy.

When you are ready, become aware of the ground beneath you and gently roll on to your side. Stay there, focus on your breath for a few moments before opening your eyes and slowly sitting up.

Breathing to relax

Focusing on the way we breathe is an integral part of relaxation. There is a yogic saying that "breath is life", but most of us never think about our breathing – we just take it for granted. Actually, our breathing changes according to how we are feeling and what we are doing. For example, when we are anxious we tend to take shallow breaths from the upper chest, which only increases anxiety. Breathing correctly from the diaphragm plays an important part in relaxation. It oxygenates the body more efficiently and prevents a build-up of carbon dioxide in the lungs.

Below I have outlined some simple breathing exercises. Take time out from your busy day to do them (perhaps at your desk or while travelling) or incorporate them into your relaxation session. If you are not used to practising conscious breathing exercises you might feel light-headed at first. The key is to take it easy and not to force the first breath.

BREATHING IN THE RELAXATION POSITION
A calmer mind and relaxed body begin with slowing the breath. Lie on your back with both knees bent, feet hip-width apart. Alternatively rest your legs on a chair, a bed or an exercise ball. You may find it useful to place an object, such as a book on your abdomen so that you can watch the way it moves up and down as you breathe. Place your hands on your lower ribcage so that your middle fingers

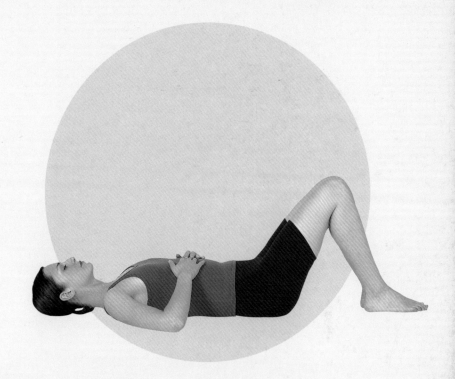

touch. Keeping your mouth closed, breathe in deeply from your diaphragm. Focus your attention on your abdomen, which should rise as you inhale. Also notice how your middle fingers separate as your ribs expand. Hold your breath for about five seconds without tensing up and then breathe out slowly through your mouth as your ribs close together again. Gradually increase the time you take to inhale and exhale so that your breathing becomes regular, rhythmic and balanced.

LATERAL THORACIC BREATHING

You can do this exercise either lying down or sitting. Wrap a long scarf or stretchband around your ribs and cross it at the front.

Hold the ends fairly tightly so that it is taut. Breathe in and allow your ribs to expand so that the scarf or band stretches. At the same time try not to allow your abdomen to rise so that you maintain a strong centre. The idea is to isolate your ribcage from your navel. As you breathe out soften the breastbone, draw the abdominals down toward the spine and gently pull the ends of the scarf or band so that you empty your lungs completely and relax your ribcage.

Meditation

Meditation, the medicine of the mind, is a way of centralizing the thoughts and calming the body. In Asia meditation has been practised for thousands of years to achieve spiritual awareness. Meditation is even more relevant today, when moments of calm are rare in our busy, stressful lives.

By becoming a master of your mind rather than a servant to it, you will discover that peace and enlightenment lie within. During meditation the hypothalamus, which is the brain's control centre for emotions as well as certain physical functions, actually expands, leading you to feel at peace. Focusing the mind on one central point also makes you become more self-aware. Practised on a regular basis, meditation should improve your ability, both mentally and physically, to cope with stress and everyday problems such as insomnia, and high blood pressure.

You can practise meditation in a group or alone. If you choose to meditate on your own, find somewhere quiet where you will not be disturbed. You may like to play some soothing music, light a candle or burn some incense to enhance the atmosphere. It is best to sit either on the floor cross-legged, or in a chair with your back well supported. Whichever position you choose make sure that you can keep your back straight without your neck becoming tense. Let your hands relax on your knees or in your lap.

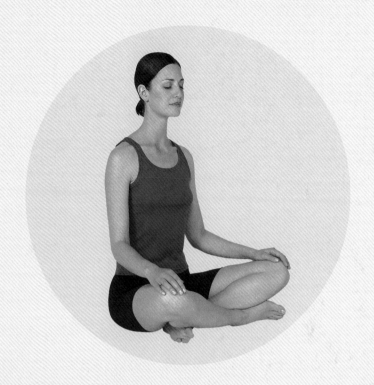

Begin by relaxing your breathing so that it becomes slower, deeper and rhythmic. Relax your mind, don't force it to concentrate – just let your thoughts drift away so that the mind stops chattering.

If you feel distracted, focus your attention on your breath. Some people find it helpful to visualize the colour light blue, which represents purity, as they breathe in, and a darker colour, such as brown, which signifies uncleanliness, as they exhale. Others prefer to focus on the flame of a candle, or to close their eyes and focus on a point within themselves, such as the heart chakra (centre).

Ridding yourself of thoughts of the past and of speculation about the future will help to create clarity in your mind and stillness in your body, but to begin with you may find that your mind wanders and thoughts keep creeping back. If this happens, don't worry – it is very difficult to empty the mind completely, especially when you are just beginning to practise meditation. However, with time and experience you will become more adept and eventually you will be able to let yourself "be" in the present moment without needing an external focus.

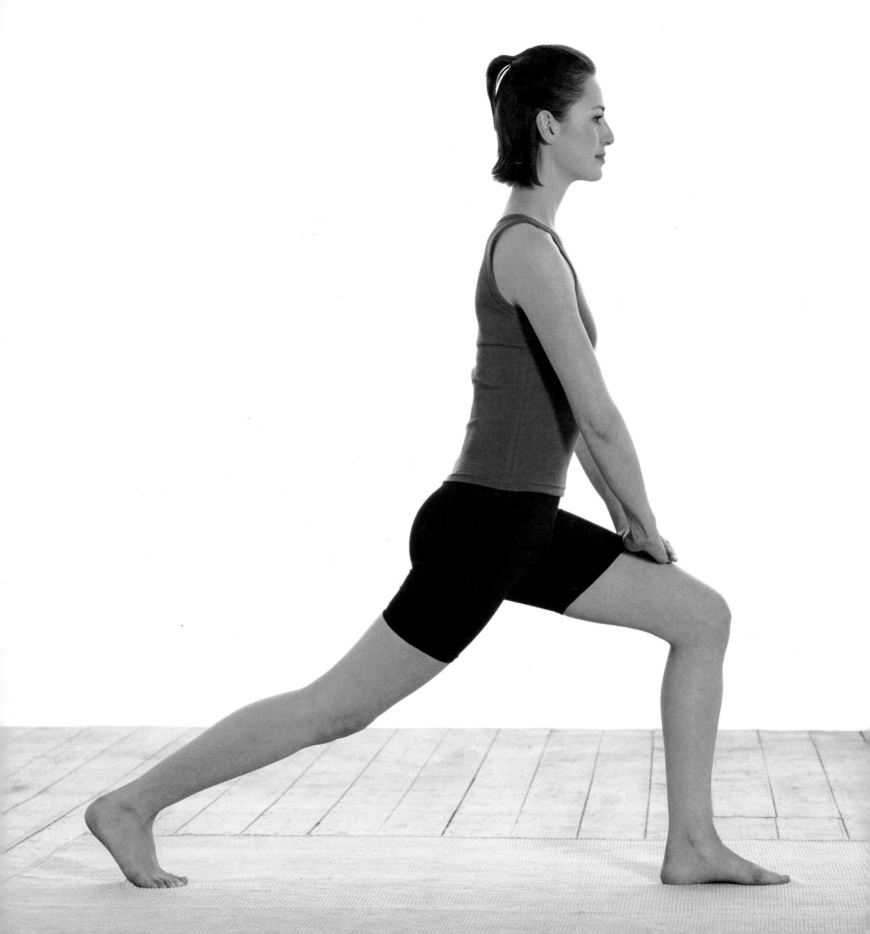

CHAPTER 5:
Easy Stretching
for Easy Sports

If you take part in sport at any level, stretching on a regular basis will improve your performance and prevent injury. Using the stretches in this book will help you to loosen the areas of your body that are tight and strengthen the areas that are weak.

In this chapter I have outlined some of the most common problems associated with certain popular sports and physical leisure activities. The key stretches for each sport or activity are illustrated, and I also suggest additional stretches which will help you to build strength and agility. If you do these stretches before or after physical activity, remember also to warm up and cool down in your usual way.

Why stretching is crucial

When we play most sports, we use a basic group of muscles, all of which require stretching in order to function properly. In addition, we use other muscles depending on which sport we are practising. For example, many sports, such as soccer and baseball involve running and the people who play them use the same core muscles. However, because the specific actions in soccer (kicking and heading a large ball) are different to those in baseball (bowling, and hitting a small ball with a bat) the specific muscles used by a soccer player will differ from those used by a baseball player.

So, when designing a stretching program for sports, it is important to take into account both the actions common to many sports and the actions specific to each sport. After analyzing the muscles used, we can gauge the patterns of muscle tightness that are likely to occur, and develop the stretches accordingly. By doing this we will achieve a higher range of mobility and prevent muscle imbalance, thereby maintaining optimal joint alignment and preventing injury.

A common problem with many sports is that they are unilateral, and therefore they develop one side of the body or one set of muscles more than the others. Golf is a prime example. When performing golf swings we rotate the spine and swing the arms the same way repeatedly. These movements place a great deal of repetitive strain on the lower back. It is therefore also important to stretch the muscles which are ignored during this movement, to avoid a physical imbalance building up in the body and to prevent injury.

If you have a coach or a fitness instructor, they will be able to advise you on the specific warm-up and cooling-down exercises that are recommended for your sport, but stretching can also help. Ideally you should stretch at the beginning of the exercise or sports session and again at the end. Stretching at the beginning helps to warm up and loosen stiff muscles, while stretching at the end helps to cool down the body and relax tired muscles. There is no way in which we can prevent all incidents that cause injury, but by doing stretching exercises we can strengthen and help prepare the muscles for activity.

Unfortunately, the level of strength and fitness of amateur sportsmen and women is often lower than their enthusiasm! This is particularly true of people over the age of fifty, who, after not exercising at all for years suddenly take up a new sport or one that they have not practised for some time. The problem is that the body's muscles weaken with age. Even healthy older people lose strength at 1–2 per cent per year, and power by 3–4 per cent per year. But the good news is that it is never too late to start exercising, playing a sport or stretching as long as you start gently.

Stretching for weight training

Weight training is useful for many people who do sport because it builds power, strength and endurance. If you use free weights, dumb bells, bar bells and so on, it is extremely important to know how to stabilize your shoulder girdle when using your arms, how to stabilize your pelvic girdle when moving your legs and how to maintain your spine in its correct postural position.

If you don't stabilize your shoulder and pelvic girdles, the muscle chains involved in lifting weights cannot operate correctly in free movement because the joints through which they transfer their strength remain unstable. The body's centre of gravity should also remain strong and neutral so that you are able to move smoothly in any direction without having to adjust your posture. The important factor is not how much weight you are able to lift, but how well you can stand and move in the correct posture while maintaining a strong core.

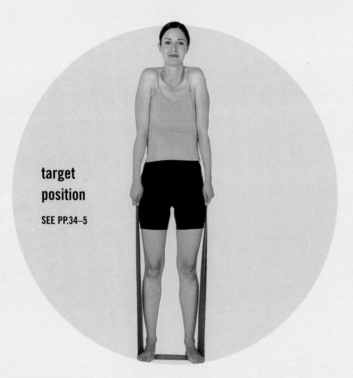

target
position

SEE PP.34–5

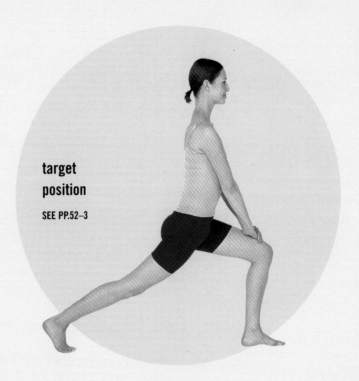

target
position

SEE PP.52–3

Stretching is the perfect companion to weight training because it keeps your body flexible as your muscles build up, becoming stronger and more powerful.

The areas of your body that will most benefit from stretching will depend on the type of weight training you are practising. For example, if you lift weights, your neck and the shoulders are probably often tight and should be stretched. But if you squat to lift bar bells, the fronts of your thighs and your hips are likely to be tight and require stretching.

As well as the key stretches shown here, I would recommend doing Spine Stretch Forward (pp.42–3), Chest Curl (pp.46–7) and Upper Chest and Shoulder Stretch (pp.36–7).

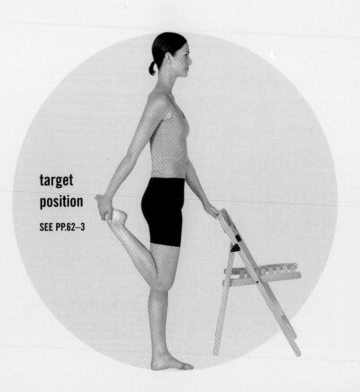

target
position

SEE PP.62–3

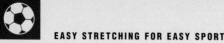

Stretching for soccer

To be a good soccer player, you need a wide range of physical skills. As well as having the ability to control the ball with your head, chest and feet, you need to be able to turn quickly and to run in fast bursts of speed. This means that you must have a wide range of movement in your joints. Stretching can help you to attain this. Kicking a football can involve a lot of hip flexion, knee extension and ankle movement. Coupled with the fact that most players seem to be either predominantly right- or left-footed, it is inevitable that they develop a unilateral imbalance. Ideally, strengthening the weaker side of the body by practising the different moves with the unfavoured side would help to restore balance, but for amateur players this is not always possible or practical. This is where stretching can be beneficial.

Which muscles of a typical soccer player are most problematic? Generally, he or she is likely to have tight hamstrings, strong dominant quadriceps (muscles in the front of

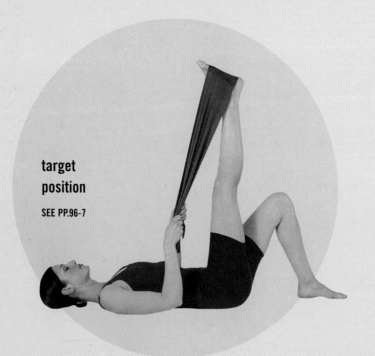

target
position
SEE PP.96-7

the thighs), very tight calf muscles, very tight hip flexors (muscles in the front of the hips), tight but sometimes weak buttock muscles and possibly, weak abdominals. Having a weak torso but strong legs can place a large amount of strain on the lower back. In addition, players who also head the ball a lot, might suffer tension in the neck and shoulder muscles and in the lower part of the spine.

As well as the key stretches depicted here, try to incorporate the following into your stretching program: Calf Stretch (pp.66–7), Front of Hip Stretch (pp.52–3), Front of Thigh Stretch (pp.62–3) and Chest Curl (pp.46–7). If you often head the ball, also include: Head Nod (pp.32–3) and Shoulder Release (pp.34–5).

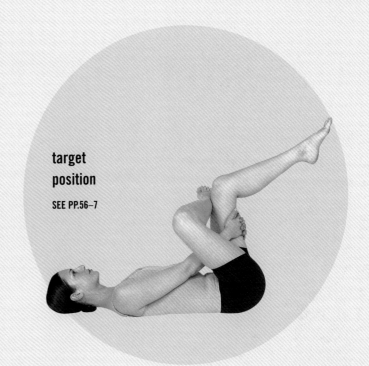

target
position

SEE PP.56–7

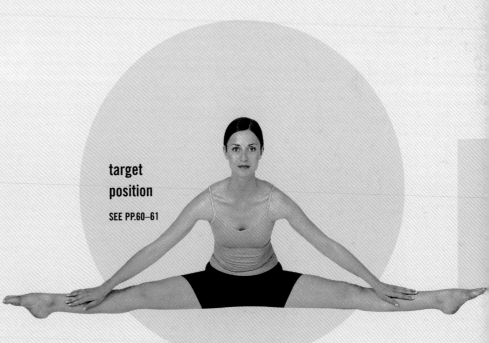

target
position

SEE PP.60–61

Stretching for running

Running or jogging is a quite different action from walking, as we are literally jumping from foot to foot, whereas when we walk we have at least one foot on the ground at all times. When we run we need to use our whole body, so if any area is stiff, we run the risk of injuring ourselves. It is particularly important to have a flexible spine and hips.

Jogging is a very popular way of keeping fit. However, if you have an imbalance in your body, such as a misaligned hip or one knee weaker than the other, this form of exercise can be a recipe for disaster.

It is a good idea to get a fitness instructor to analyze the way you run before you start doing it regularly. Also make sure that you buy a pair of good-quality running shoes. You then need to stretch and strengthen the muscles of your feet so that they can work properly inside the shoes. For this purpose, the Foot and Ankle Stretch (pp.68–9), using the stretchband around your foot or simply

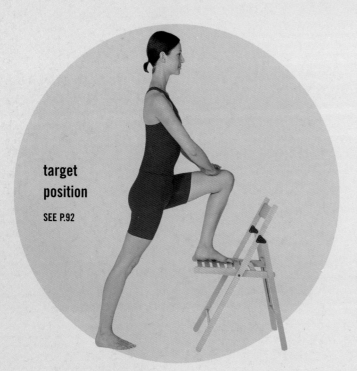

target position

SEE P.92

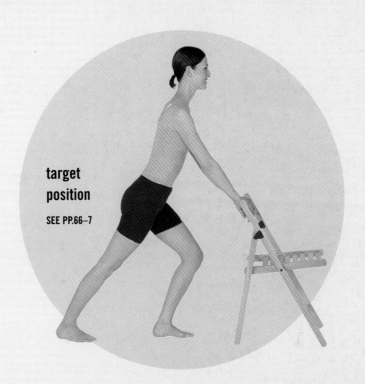

target
position
SEE PP.66–7

rising up onto the balls of your feet, are

particularly effective.

Running tends to overuse the following

muscles: the quadriceps (at the front of the

thighs) the hamstrings, calves and shins. The

hip flexors (at the front of the hips) are also

usually very tight in runners. Often, with the

additional swinging movement of the arms,

runners can also build up tension in the neck

and shoulders.

In addition to the key stretches shown

here, I would suggest doing Outer Thigh Stretch

(pp.64–5), Hamstring Stretch (pp.58–9), Front

of Thigh Stretch (pp.62–3), and, if you run on

concrete (which stresses the lower spine),

Spine Stretch Forward (pp.42–3).

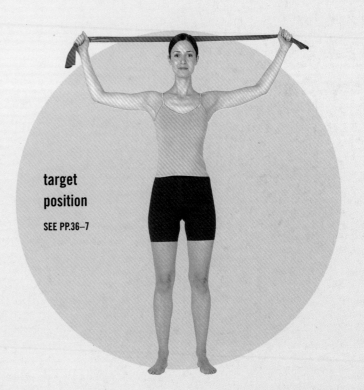

target
position
SEE PP.36–7

Stretching for racquet sports

Racquet sports, such as tennis, squash and badminton tend to use one side of the body more than the other, involving repetitive movements with the arm and the shoulder, as well as rotation of the trunk. These movements can build up a muscular imbalance in the body, which can be partly redressed by stretching.

Before you start playing a racquet sport, it is important to build strength by stretching the upper body and shoulders. If there is not enough strength in these areas, other muscles will compensate, which could cause injury.

In addition to the stretches shown here, I recommend that you practise some wrist extensions. If you are right-handed, hold your right arm; if you are left-handed, hold your left arm. Bend your wrist so that your fingers point down to the floor. Keep your elbow locked. This is an important stretch to alleviate tennis elbow, a condition in which the muscles most commonly affected are the wrist extensors.

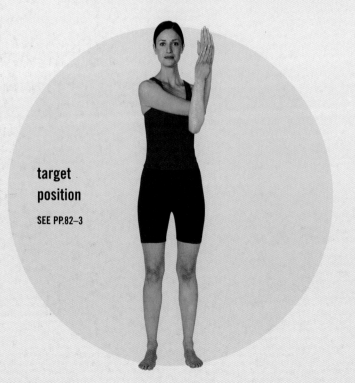

target position

SEE PP.82–3

You could also try placing the back of your hand against a wall and leaning on it slightly, keeping your elbow locked.

Other stretches that are effective for racquet sports players are Head Tilt (pp.30–31), Head Nod (pp.32–3), Shoulder Release (pp.34–5), Buttock Stretch (pp.56–7), Hamstring Stretch (pp.58–9), Front of Thigh Stretch (pp.62–3), Calf Stretch (pp.66–7) and Waist Stretch (pp.50–51).

If you are incorporating stretches into your playing session, remember to warm-up first, *then* stretch. Carefully run through your strokes without a ball or shuttlecock for a couple of minutes before starting your game. Then stretch again when you've finished.

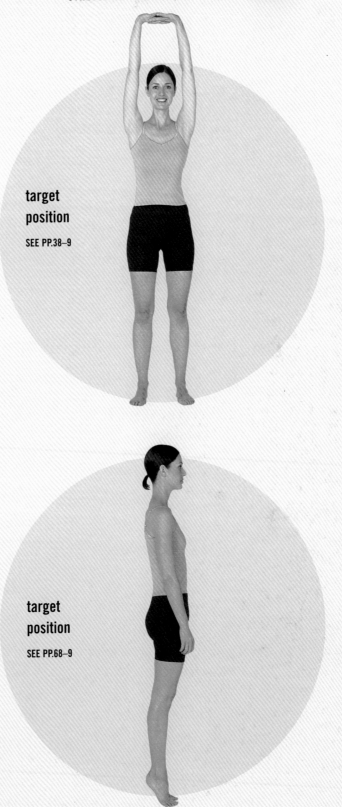

target
position
SEE PP.38–9

target
position
SEE PP.68–9

Stretching for dance and aerobics

People who dance or do aerobics as leisure activities require cardiovascular fitness as well as strength and flexibility. Because these activities involve much movement of the arms and legs, the abdominal muscles are often overlooked. Whatever form of dance or aerobics you do, always try to maintain a strong abdominal centre, which will help your limbs to move freely and safely and will also protect your spine.

When dancing or performing aerobics we breathe quickly and shallowly. For this reason many dancers and aerobics teachers tend to be very tight across the upper chest and back. It is therefore beneficial to focus on deepening and slowing your breath when you perform stretches – and you should do so also both before and after your class.

Common problems associated with dance and aerobics include: knee injuries, foot and ankle problems (particularly with the Achilles tendon, if you jump a lot), and back tightness.

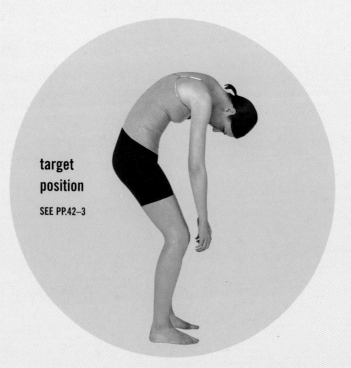

target
position
SEE PP.42–3

In addition to the three stretches suggested here you could also include Upper Chest and Shoulder Stretch (pp.36–7), Spine Stretch Back (pp.44–5), Chest Curl (pp.46–7), Hamstring Stretch (pp.58–9) and Foot and Ankle Stretch (pp.68–9).

Dance and aerobics place a great deal of strain on the joints, which can cause arthritis or osteoporosis later in life. If you find it hard to keep dancing or doing aerobics as you get older, and you decide to give them up, don't stop stretching altogether. Instead, just stretch more gently, because your body is used to making those movements and the muscle memory remains. By continuing to stretch you will keep your joints lubricated and supple.

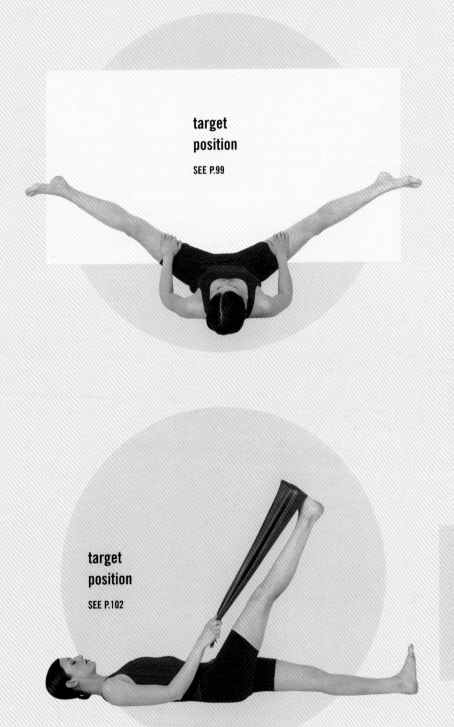

target
position

SEE P.99

target
position

SEE P.102

Stretching for golf

Golf is another sport in which we tend to use one side of our body more than the other. A good player performs a typical golf swing by angling the body slightly forward from the hips, which together with the knees are slightly flexed. After rotating the trunk to the right or left to lift the golf club over the shoulder, it is the ability to twist the whole spine that is the hallmark of a good swing. Because driving and chipping the ball require you to move your body repeatedly in the same direction, in an action that places strain on your lower spine, it is important to have a flexible spine and supple hips. You also need to have strong abdominal muscles to support your spine throughout the game. Even just carrying the golf clubs around the course can place a tremendous strain on your back and shoulders.

This means that the areas of the body most vulnerable and prone to injury in this sport are the lower spine, the hips, the neck, the shoulders and the forearms.

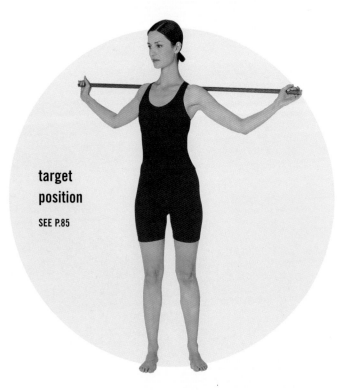

target
position

SEE P.85

Stretching can be of real benefit to strengthen the spine and to make both the spine and the hips more flexible. It is particularly important to stretch often if you are a golfer who spends long periods sitting, say working at a desk, which can cause tension and stiffness in your shoulders and upper back.

In addition to the key stretches shown here, it would be beneficial to include the following in your stretching routine: Upper Chest and Shoulder Stretch (pp.36–7), both Head Tilt (pp.30–31) and Head Nod (pp.32–3), Spine Stretch Forward (pp.42–3) and Chest Curl (pp.46–7) for strengthening your abdominal muscles.

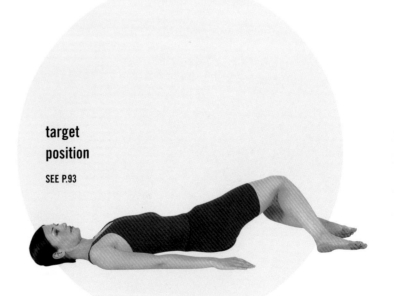

target
position

SEE P.81

target
position

SEE P.93

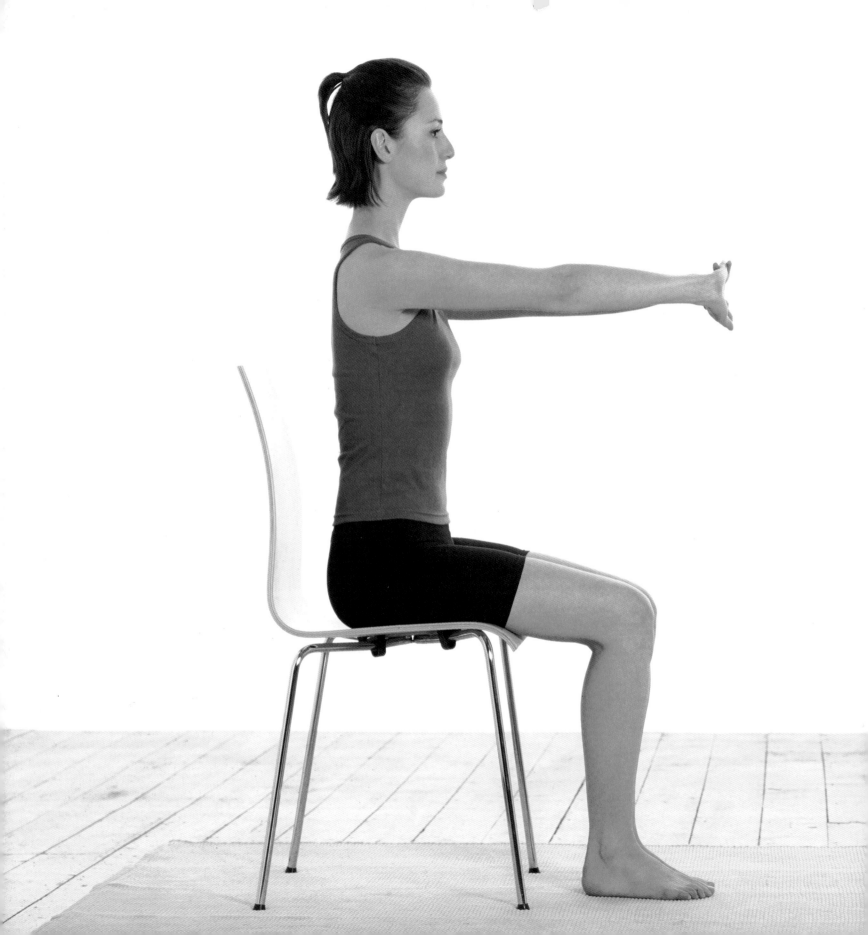

CHAPTER 6:
Easy Stretching
for Everyday Life

The unrelenting pace of modern life inevitably take its toll on us,
causing us physical and/or emotional stress. In this chapter I outline
some common, everyday movements – actions that we perform regularly
at home and at work, such as sitting, lifting and carrying – and advise
how to accomplish them correctly and improve postural alignment.

For those of you who spend time at a desk or in front of a computer,
there are a few extra stretches in addition to those in Chapters 2 and 3.
A short section on travel illuminates the effects that the various types
of transport have on our bodies, and suggests stretches to counteract
any ill effects we might suffer.

When deciding which stretches to do, take into account your average
day – the activities and movements you tend to repeat. Then use this
information to create a stretching routine that fits in with your lifestyle.

An antidote to modern lifestyles

If we strain or use our bodies awkwardly, we can create stress and tension in our muscles simply by carrying out everyday tasks. Day in, day out we repeat the same incorrect movements, oblivious to the continual build-up of muscular tension, until eventually our bodies stiffen up completely in a kind of muscular rigor mortis. Sometimes we are so unaware of this deterioration that it is only when certain movements become very uncomfortable or even painful, that we realize we must do something about our physical state. If only we had known that just by doing a little stretching each day we could have prevented so much muscular tension from accumulating.

Another common problem caused by our sedentary modern lifestyle is back pain. Because many of us sit at desks all day, our spines suffer far more compression than they would if we were standing. The problem is exacerbated if we slouch. Pressure on the discs also increases as we get older.

The key to avoiding back problems is to be aware of the way you sit. Ideally your back should be straight, without being too rigid, Try to keep your shoulders down and your abdominal muscles pulled in to help flatten your lower back into the chair. Also, be careful when getting in and out of your chair, as this can place a huge strain on your lower back. Move your buttocks to the edge of the seat first, keeping your back straight. Then, keeping your abdominals strong, use your thigh muscles and arms to help you elevate your body,

Lifting and carrying are also potentially dangerous for the back, neck and shoulders. Never bend from the waist – instead aim to bend at the hips and knees. When you pick up an object, try to keep it as close to your body as possible, and again be aware of using your core strength to help you. Use the same technique to put an object down. When lifting or carrying something, particularly if it is heavy, try to distribute the weight equally on both sides of your body to prevent straining one side.

If you are a keen gardener, try to stretch before you start to prepare your body for the physical work of weeding, digging, planting and so on. Then stretch again when you have finished to relax your tired muscles.

It might be helpful to make a note of and analyze the type of movements you perform in an average week. For example, do you sit for long periods? Does your work involve bending, reaching or standing? Once you recognize the most likely areas of tightness in your body, you can concentrate on stretching them regularly to release the tension.

Always listen to your body. When it tells you that it needs to stretch, stretch it; but when it feels that it needs to relax, rest it.

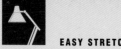

Desk stretches

Both adults who work in offices, and children in school can suffer from bad posture when sitting at a desk or table, especially if they frequently use computers. Bad posture is one of the main causes of on-going back, neck and shoulder problems.

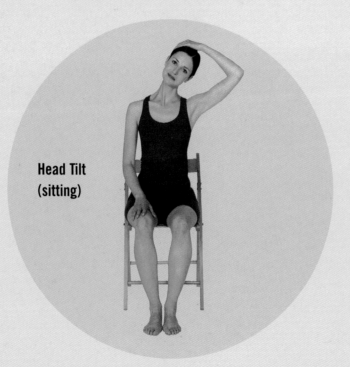

Head Tilt
(sitting)

Here are a few simple stretches that target the areas of the body most prone to tension when we sit at a desk or a table.

NECK (Head Tilt)

This is the same as the modified Head Tilt (p.76), only you remain seated. Sit tall with your back straight and your abdominals strong. Inhale. As you exhale tilt your head toward your left shoulder and let your right shoulder drop. Now repeat the movement, this time tilting your head toward your right shoulder and dropping your left shoulder.

Another stretch which is very effective for releasing tension at the top of the neck, is to move your head as if you are one of those

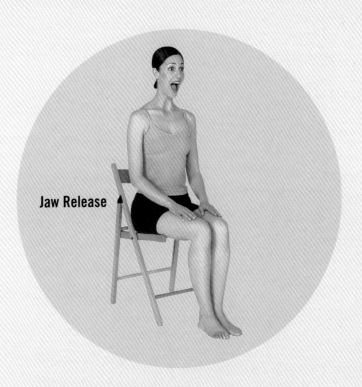

Jaw Release

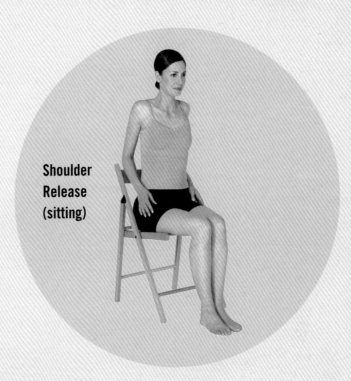

Shoulder
Release
(sitting)

nodding dogs that people have in the back of
their car. Make tiny nodding movements
so that your chin only drops about an inch
forward. Do a few nods with your eyes closed,
to give your eyes a rest.

FACE (Jaw Release)

Open your mouth as wide as possible and in
this position try to smile slightly, then relax
your mouth. This exercise releases any tension
caused by clenching or grinding the teeth.

You can also try relaxing your mouth while
keeping it slightly open and then sliding
your jaw from side to side.

SHOULDERS (Shoulder Release)

Inhale and lift your shoulders up toward your
ears. Exhale and let them slide down into your
back. You can try this with both shoulders
at the same time, or one at a time or even
incorporating a circular movement in either
a forward or backward direction.

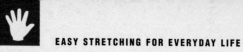

Hands and Fingers

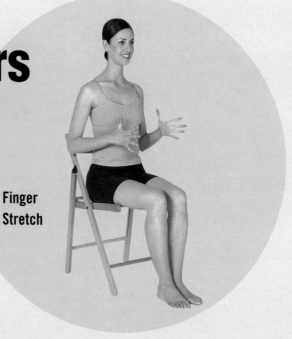

Finger Stretch

To give your fingers a break from keyboard work, alternate between clenching your fingers tightly and stretching and separating them. Repeat 10 to 20 times.

Next, we have a modified version of the Upper Arm and Shoulder Pull (see pp.38–9). Push your office chair away from your desk, so that you have enough space to stretch your arms out in front of you without touching your computer.

Sit with a straight back and then interlace your fingers with your palms facing away from you and your arms extended forward. You could also include the second modified stretch (p.83) by pulling your arm across your body.

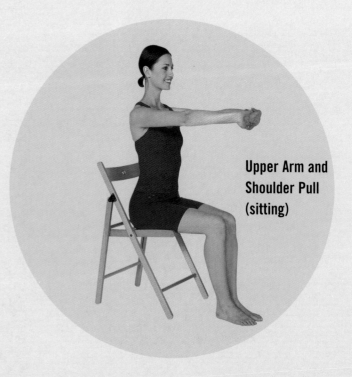

Upper Arm and Shoulder Pull (sitting)

Legs and Feet

Think of your feet as your body's foundations and keep them moving to increase your circulation. Getting up and walking around is an ideal way of stretching your legs and feet. Otherwise, simply practise both the modified exercises in Chapter 3 – Calf Stretch (p.102) and Foot and Ankle Stretch (p.103). (You can easily do the point and flex exercise without using a stretchband.) About 5 to 10 stretches with each leg will work the muscles of the feet and lower leg and improve your circulation.

You can also do the Foot and Ankle Stretch (pp.68–9) sitting in a chair. Remove your shoes and alternate between rising up on to the balls of your feet and lowering your heels back down to the floor.

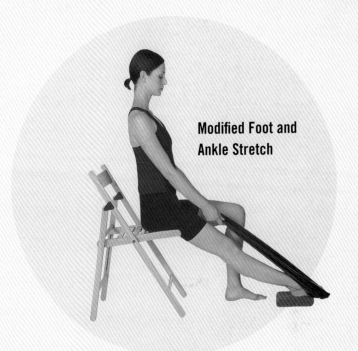

Modified Foot and
Ankle Stretch

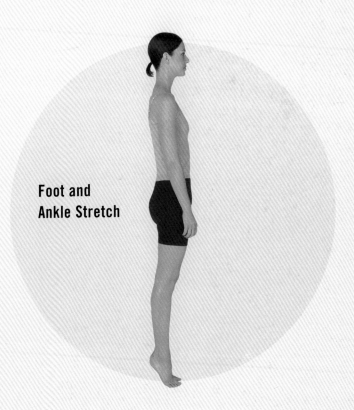

Foot and
Ankle Stretch

Car and train stretches

Travelling by car, especially if you are the driver, aggravates the back and stiffens the legs, particularly if you have to remain in one position for long periods of time. If you are driving through heavy traffic or you are stuck in a traffic jam, you have to keep using the pedals, changing gear and braking, all actions that put increased pressure on your legs and hips. When you do find yourself stuck in a traffic jam or even waiting for the traffic lights to turn green, use the time to do some neck stretches or shoulder shrugs. You can also practise pulling in your abdominal muscles and lifting your pelvic floor muscles. If you are a passenger, you can do these exercises at any time. Whether you are the driver or a passenger never drive for too long without stopping to take a break and walk around to stretch your legs.

In addition to the stretches mentioned above, which you can do inside the car, you could practise the modified Front of Hip

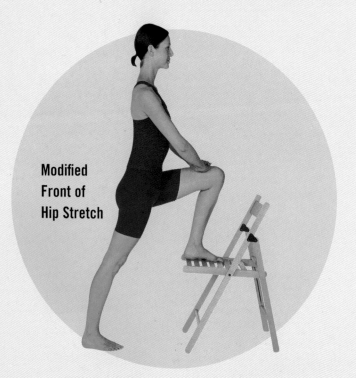

Modified Front of Hip Stretch

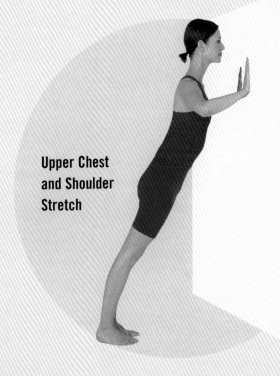

Upper Chest and Shoulder Stretch

Stretch (see p.92). Simply place one leg up on the car wing and lean forward to stretch the opposite hip. Or try the Calf Stretch (see pp.66–7) leaning on the car instead of holding on to a chair.

Travelling by train is far more back-friendly than travelling by car, because you are free to move around whenever you like. You can relax, sleep, listen to music or read. It is important to be aware of the position of your head. Unfortunately the headrests are not adjustable on trains and this can often cause the head to lean forward from the neck. To prevent tension from building up in your neck, simply rest your head back against the headrest and make a small figure of eight shape with the tip of your nose. Do this a few times in one direction and then in reverse.

As there are so many doorways in a train, it is easy to use them to lean against to stretch the upper chest and shoulders. Try the third modified position for the Upper Chest and Shoulder Stretch (p.81) with your arms in the doorway leaning slightly forward. You could also do foot rises (see pp.68–9) holding on to the doorway, or the neck and shoulder exercises suggested for car drivers and passengers.

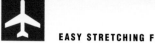
Airplane stretches

Travelling by airplane, especially on long-haul flights, can be both mentally and physically stressful. Many people suffer from a slight fear of flying, which can make their body full of tension until they arrive at their destination. During a flight, you often have to sit for long periods without space to stretch your legs or back, which can restrict your circulation and increase your risk of DVT (deep vein thrombosis). For this reason it is good to get yourself a seat next to the aisle, whenever possible, so that you can walk up and down the cabin frequently.

It is wise to take some exercise, such as walking, running or swimming before flying. During the flight you could try wearing compression hosiery, which provides extra support for the leg veins to aid circulation and reduces the build-up of excess fluid. Also, keep moving your head, neck and shoulders.

As the ankles are prone to swelling during travel it is important to keep your feet and

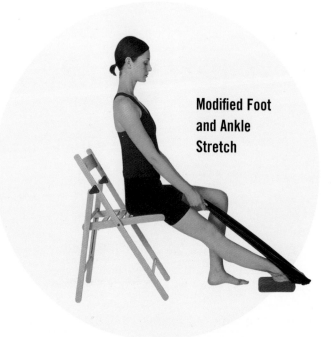

Modified Foot and Ankle Stretch

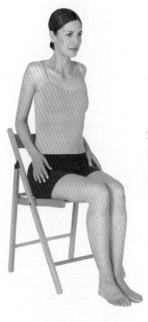

**Shoulder
Release
(sitting)**

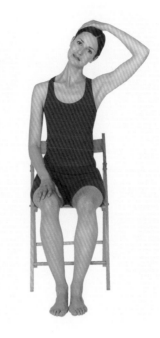

**Head Tilt
(sitting)**

ankles moving. If you are sitting in an inside seat and getting out to walk up the aisle regularly involves disturbing fellow passengers, you can always exercise your legs while remaining seated. An easy exercise to do from your seat is to lift one heel off the floor, keeping your weight on the ball of your foot and toes. Alternate feet in this movement, so that as one heel lowers the other lifts up. It is easier to do this exercise if you take off your shoes first.

Another exercise you may like to try is to lift one thigh off the seat and clasp both hands under it for support. Circle the ankle of the elevated leg ten times to the right and ten times to the left. Then, repeat the exercise with the other leg.

When you finally reach your destination, stretch your back – try Spine Stretch Forward (pp.42–3) and Spine Stretch Back (pp.44–5). If your legs have swollen during the flight, lie with them elevated to reduce the swelling.

Bibliography

Anderson, Bob *Stretching*, Shelter Publications (Bolinas, California, USA), 2000

Blakey, W. Paul *Stretching Without Pain*, Bibliotek Books (Stafford, UK), 1994 and Twin Eagles Publishing (Sechelt, Canada), 1995

Crowther, Ann *Pilates for You*, Duncan Baird Publishers (London), 2003 and *Total Pilates*, Thorsons (Boston), 2003

Mitchell, Emma *Energy Exercises* Duncan Baird Publishers (London), and Celestial Arts, an imprint of Tenspeed (Berkeley, California, USA), 2000

Norris, Christopher *The Complete Guide to Stretching*, A & C Black (London), 2000

Rosser, Mo *Body Fitness and Exercise: Basic Theory and Practice for Therapists*, Hodder and Stoughton (London), 1995

Smith, Karen *Body & Soul: A Woman's Guide to Staying Young*, Kyle Cathie (London), 1998

Summers, Neil *The Art of Backstretching*, Enanef Press (Dorking, Surrey, UK), 2000

Thompson, Ken *The Movement Book*, Bibliotek Books (Stafford, Staffordshire, UK), 1996

Tobias, Maxine and Sullivan, John Patrick *The Complete Stretching Book*, Dorling Kindersley (London) and Knopf (New York), 1992

Walker, Brad *The Stretching Handbook*, Walkerbout Health (Robina, Queensland, Australia), 1997

Index

Acknowledgments

My thanks to photographer Matthew Ward for
all his patience during the photo shoots; to our
model, Poppy Armitage, for endless hours of
stretching; to Ursula Hageli for typing up my
text; and to Naina Patel BSc. (Hons), NCSP
for all her help and advice.

Karen Smith can be found at www.karensmithpilates.com